UROLOGIC CLINICS
OF NORTH AMERICA

Pelvic Neuromodulation

GUEST EDITOR
Firouz Daneshgari, MD

CONSULTING EDITOR
Martin I. Resnick, MD

February 2005 • Volume 32 • Number 1

SAUNDERS

An Imprint of Elsevier, Inc.
PHILADELPHIA   LONDON   TORONTO   MONTREAL   SYDNEY   TOKYO

W.B. SAUNDERS COMPANY

A Division of Elsevier Inc.

The Curtis Center • Independence Square West • Philadelphia, Pennsylvania 19106

http://www.theclinics.com

THE UROLOGIC CLINICS OF NORTH AMERICA
February 2005
Editor: Catherine Bewick

Volume 32, Number 1
ISSN 0094-0143
ISBN 1-4160-2800-5

Reprints. For copies of 100 or more, of articles in this publication, please contact the Commercial Reprints Department, Elsevier Inc., 360 Park Avenue South, New York, New York 10010-1710. Tel.: (212) 633-3813, Fax: (212) 462-1935, e-mail: reprints@elsevier.com.

The ideas and opinions expressed in *The Urologic Clinics of North America* do not necessarily reflect those of the Publisher. The Publisher does not assume any responsibility for any injury and/or damage to persons or property arising out of or related to any use of the material contained in this periodical. The reader is advised to check the appropriate medical literature and the product information currently provided by the manufacturer of each drug to be administered to verify the dosage, the method and duration of administration, or contraindications. It is the responsibility of the treating physician or other health care professional, relying on independent experience and knowledge of the patient, to determine drug dosages and the best treatment for the patient. Mention of any product in this issue should not be construed as endorsement by the contributors, editors, or the Publisher of the product or manufacturers' claims.

The Urologic Clinics of North America (ISSN 0094-0143) is published quarterly by W.B. Saunders Company. Corporate and editorial offices: The Curtis Center, Independence Square West, Philadelphia, PA 19106-3399. Accounting and circulation offices: 6277 Sea Harbor Drive, Orlando, FL 32887-4800. Periodicals postage paid at Orlando, FL 32862, and additional mailing offices. Subscription prices are $195.00 per year (US individuals), $307.00 per year (US institutions), $225.00 per year (Canadian individuals), $371.00 per year (Canadian institutions), $260.00 per year (foreign individuals), and $371.00 per year (foreign institutions). Foreign air speed delivery is included in all *Clinics* subscription prices. All prices are subject to change without notice. POSTMASTER: Send address changes to *The Urologic Clinics of North America*, W.B. Saunders Company, Periodicals Fulfillment, Orlando, FL 32887-4800. **Customer Service: 1-800-654-2452 (US). From outside the US, call 1-407-345-4000.**

The Urologic Clinics of North America is covered in *Index Medicus*, *Excerpta Medica*, *Current Contents/Clinical Medicine*, *Science Citation Index*, and *ISI/BIOMED*.

Printed in the United States of America.

CONSULTING EDITOR

MARTIN I. RESNICK, MD, Lester Persky Professor and Chairman, Department of Urology, Case Western Reserve University, School of Medicine/University Hospitals, Cleveland, Ohio

GUEST EDITOR

FIROUZ DANESHGARI, MD, Director, Center for Female Pelvic Medicine & Reconstructive Surgery, The Cleveland Clinic Foundation, Glickman Urological Institute, Cleveland, Ohio

CONTRIBUTORS

PAUL ABRAMS, MD, Professor of Urology, Bristol Urological Institute, Southmead Hospital, Bristol, United Kingdom

AHMAD H. BANI-HANI, MD, Resident, Department of Urology, Mayo Graduate School of Medicine, Rochester, Minnesota

ANDREW J. BERNSTEIN, MD, Department of Urology, William Beaumont Hospital, Royal Oak, Michigan

J.L.H.R. BOSCH, MD, PhD, Professor and Chairman, Department of Urology, University Medical Center Utrecht, Utrecht, The Netherlands

TOBY C. CHAI, MD, FACS, Associate Professor, Division of Urology, University of Maryland School of Medicine, Baltimore, Maryland

MICHAEL B. CHANCELLOR, MD, Professor of Urology, Department of Urology, University of Pittsburgh School of Medicine, Pittsburgh, Pennsylvania

MATTHEW R. COOPERBERG, MD, MPH, Resident, Department of Urology, University of California, San Francisco, California

FIROUZ DANESHGARI, MD, Director, Center for Female Pelvic Medicine & Reconstructive Surgery, The Cleveland Clinic Foundation, Glickman Urological Institute, Cleveland, Ohio

R.A. DE BIE, MD, PhD, Department of Epidemiology, Maastricht University Hospital, Maastricht, The Netherlands.

MOHAMED ELKELINI, MD, Research Fellow, Division of Urology, Toronto Western Hospital, University Health Network, University of Toronto, Toronto, Ontario, Canada

THOMAS FANDEL, MD, Research Fellow, Department of Urology, University of California School of Medicine, San Francisco, California

TARA L. FRENKL, MD, MPH, Fellow, Female Pelvic Medicine and Reconstructive Surgery, The Cleveland Clinic Foundation, Glickman Urological Institute, Cleveland, Ohio

MAGDY M. HASSOUNA, MD, PhD, FRCSC, FACS, Associate Professor, Division of Urology, Toronto Western Hospital, University Health Network, University of Toronto, Toronto, Ontario, Canada

ADONIS HIJAZ, MD, Clinical Fellow, Female Pelvic Medicine & Reconstructive Surgery, The Cleveland Clinic Foundation, Glickman Urological Institute, Cleveland, Ohio

MICHAEL E.D. JARRETT, MA, MRCS, Research Fellow, Boundary House, Little Milton, United Kingdom

WENDY W. LENG, MD, Assistant Professor of Urology, Department of Urology, University of Pittsburgh School of Medicine, Pittsburgh, Pennsylvania

M. LOUIS MOY, MD, Assistant Professor, Department of Urology, University of Pennsylvania, Philadelphia, Pennsylvania

KENNETH M. PETERS, MD, Department of Urology, William Beaumont Hospital, Royal Oak, Michigan

RAYMOND R. RACKLEY, MD, Co-Section Head, Section of Voiding Dysfunction and Female Urology, The Cleveland Clinic Foundation, Glickman Urological Institute, Cleveland, Ohio

YURI E. REINBERG, MD, Attending Pediatric Urologist, Pediatric Surgical Associates, Minneapolis, Minnesota; and Assistant Professor, Department of Urology, Mayo Clinic, Rochester, Minnesota

W.A. SCHEEPENS, MD, PhD, Department of Urology, Maastricht University Hospital, Maastricht, The Netherlands

STEVEN W. SIEGEL, MD, Director, Center for Continence Care, Metropolitan Urologic Specialists, St. Paul, Minnesota

MARSHALL L. STOLLER, MD, Professor, Department of Urology, University of California, San Francisco, California

EMIL A. TANAGHO, MD, Professor, Department of Urology, University of California School of Medicine, San Francisco, California

DAVID R. VANDERSTEEN, MD, Attending Pediatric Urologist, Pediatric Surgical Associates, Minneapolis, Minnesota; and Assistant Professor, Department of Urology, Mayo Clinic, Rochester, Minnesota

PH. E.V. VAN KERREBROECK, MD, PhD, Department of Urology, Maastricht University Hospital, Maastricht, The Netherlands

SANDIP VASAVADA, MD, Co-Section Head, Section of Voiding Dysfunction and Female Urology, The Cleveland Clinic Foundation, Glickman Urological Institute, Cleveland, Ohio

E.H.J. WEIL, MD, PhD, Department of Urology, Maastricht University Hospital, Maastricht, The Netherlands

CONTENTS

gram. A successful trial stimulation remains the best indicator for patient selection, and should be used as a routine diagnostic test among patients who have chronic, life-altering voiding complaints that cannot be resolved adequately by medications or behavioral interventions.

Sacral neurostimulation is an accepted form of therapy for voiding dysfunction. Multiple modifications in surgical techniques have resulted in a minimally invasive procedure. These modifications include implantation of pulse generator in buttock area, fluoroscopic guidance for S3 lead implantation, percutaneous methodology for S3 lead implantation, development of the tined S3 lead, and use of the staged implantation. These modifications have decreased surgical time, increased acceptance of this therapy among surgeons and patients, and increased overall efficacy and efficiency of S3 stimulation therapy.

Neuromodulation is becoming a part of the clinical armamentarium for treatment of a variety of lower urinary tract conditions. Its increased usage stems from the needs of patients who have exhausted all other therapeutic options. Currently, neuromodulation may consist of the use of nerve stimulation and injectable therapies. This article concentrates on nerve stimulation.

Sacral nerve modulation has become an established modality for treatment of voiding dysfunction. This article presents a review of the use of sacral neuromodulation as a treatment option in patients with voiding dysfunction. The first part discusses the different aspects of neuromodulation. The second part presents experience in neuromodulation use in Canada, including a review of the results of basic research done at University of Toronto, in addition to the long-term results in patients with sacral neuromodulation.

This article discusses the European experience with bilateral sacral neuromodulation in patients who have chronic lower urinary tract dysfunction.

Neuromodulation to treat voiding dysfunction has been studied for decades. Since its inception, widespread use for approved conditions has led to incidental improvements in other areas. Research is ongoing to channel the potential of neuromodulation into other applications. The major frontiers for sacral neuromodulation in adults are interstitial cystitis and chronic pain syndromes, neurogenic bladder from spinal cord injury, fecal incontinence and constipation, and erectile dysfunction. Projects are ongoing studying the efficacy of neuromodulation in children with voiding dysfunction.

GOAL STATEMENT

The goal of *Urologic Clinics of North America* is to keep practicing urologists and urology residents up to date with current clinical practice in urology by providing timely articles reviewing the state of the art in patient care.

ACCREDITATION

The *Urologic Clinics of North America* is planned and implemented in accordance with the Essential Areas and Policies of the Accreditation Council for Continuing Medical Education (ACCME) through the joint sponsorship of the University of Virginia School of Medicine and W. B. Saunders Company. The University of Virginia School of Medicine is accredited by the ACCME to provide continuing medical education for physicians.

The University of Virginia School of Medicine designates this educational activity for a maximum of 60 category 1 credits per year, 15 category 1 credits per issue, toward the AMA Physician's Recognition Award. Each physician should claim only those credits that he/she actually spent in the activity.

The American Medical Association has determined that physicians not licensed in the US who participate in this CME activity are eligible for AMA PRA category 1 credit.

Category 1 credit can be earned by reading the text material, taking the CME examination online at http://www.theclinics.com/home/cme, and completing the evaluation. After taking the test, you will be required to review any and all incorrect answers. Following completion of the test and evaluation, your credit will be awarded and you may print your certificate.

FACULTY DISCLOSURE

As a provider accredited by the Accreditation Council for Continuing Medical Education (ACCME), the Office of Continuing Medical Education of the University of Virginia School of Medicine must ensure balance, independence, objectivity, and scientific rigor in all its individually sponsored or jointly sponsored educational activities. All authors/editors participating in a sponsored activity are expected to disclose to the readers any significant financial interest or other relationship (1) with the manufacturer(s) of any commercial product(s) and/or provider(s) of commercial services discussed in an educational presentation and (2) with any commercial supporters of the activity (significant financial interest or other relationship can include such things as grants or research support, employee, consultant, stock holder, member of speakers bureau, etc.) The intent of this disclosure is not to prevent authors/editors with a significant financial or other relationship from writing an article, but rather to provide readers with information on which they can make their own judgments. It remains for the readers to determine whether the author's/editor's interest or relationships may influence the article with regard to exposition or conclusion.

The authors/editors listed below have identified no professional or financial affiliations related to their presentation:
Ahmad H. Bani-Hani, MD; Andrew J. Bernstein, MD; Catherine Bewick, Acquisitions Editor; Toby C. Chai, MD, FACS; Matthew R. Copperberg, MD, MPH; Firouz Daneshgari, MD; Mohamed Elkelini, MD; Thomas Fandel, MD; Tara L. Frenkl, MD, MPH; Adonis Hijaz, MD; Magdy M. Hassouna, MD, PhD: Michael E. D. Jarrett, MA, MRCS; Wendy W. Leng, MD; M. Louise Moy, MD; Yuri E. Reinberg, MD; Martin J. Resnick, MD; and, Emil A. Tanagho, MD.

The authors/editors listed below have identified the following professional or financial affiliations related to their article:
J. L. H. R. Bosch, MD, PhD is investigator and consultant for advanced bionics the manufacturer of the bion device.
R. A. de Bie; W A. Scheepens; Philip E. V. van Kerrebroeck, MD, PhD; and, **E. H. J. Weil** have disclosed that they are investigators for Medtronic.
Kenneth M. Peters, MD is a consultant and investigator for Advanced Bionics, and a consultant and proctor for Medtronic Corporation.
Steven W. Siegel, MD is a clinical researcher, consultant, lecturer, and proctor for Medtronic Corporation.
Marshall L. Stoller, MD developed the SANS percutaneous system that will potentially be commercially available in the next year.
Sandip Vasavada, MD is a preceptor for Medtronic Corporation.

Disclosure of Discussion of non-FDA approved uses for pharmaceutical products and/or medical devices: The University of Virginia School of Medicine, as an ACCME provider, requires that all faculty presenters identify and disclose any "off label" uses for pharmaceutical and medical device products. The University of Virginia School of Medicine recommends that each physician fully review all the available data on new products or procedures prior to instituting them with patients.

The following authors will be discussing the off-label use of the following pharmaceutical or medical device products:
Andrew J. Bernstein, MD will the use of sacral neuromodulation for interstitial cystitis, chronic pain syndromes (pelvic pain, prostadyma, epidiymo-orchalgia, vulvodynia), neurogenic bladder in spinal cord injury, fecal incontinence/constipation, erectile dysfuntion, migraine headaches, and, chronic angina pectoris.
Firouz Daneshgari, MD will discuss the treatment of interstitial cystitis, pelvic pain, neurogenic bladder.
R. A. de Bie; W A. Scheepens; Philip E. V. van Kerrebroeck, MD, PhD; and, E. H. J. Weil Will discuss the use of the Medtronic Interstim device for bilateral sacral nerve stimulation.
Tara L. Frenkl, MD, MPH will discuss the use of Botulinum toxin for overactive bladder, interstitial cystitis, detrusor sphincter dysynergia, and pelvic pain.
Kenneth M. Peters, MD will discuss the treatment of interstitial cystitis, chronic pain syndromes, neurogenic bladder, fecal incontinence/constipation, erectile dysfunction, migraine headaches, chronic angina pectoris.
Yuri E. Reinberg, MD will discuss the use of Interstim in children.

The authors/editors listed below have not provided disclosure or off-label information:
Paul Abrams, MD; Michael B. Chancellor, MD; Raymond R. Rackley, MD; and, David R. Vandersteen, MD.

TO ENROLL

To enroll in the Urologic Clinics of North America Continuing Medical Education program, call customer service at 1-800-654-2452 or visit us online at www.theclinics.com/home/cme. The CME program is available to subscribers for an additional fee of $165.00

FORTHCOMING ISSUES

RECENT ISSUES

THE CLINICS ARE NOW AVAILABLE ONLINE!

Access your subscription at:
http://www.theclinics.com

UROLOGIC
CLINICS
of North America

Urol Clin N Am 32 (2005) xi

Foreword

Pelvic Neuromodulation

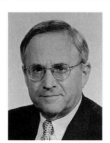

Martin I. Resnick, MD
Consulting Editor

Though the concept may be old, the term *neuromodulation* is new, and it is one that promises to not only become used with increasing frequency but whose principles will greatly impact the practice of urology and, on a wider perspective, the practice of medicine. The idea of stimulating nerves to improve bodily functions and patient symptoms most certainly has the potential of greatly benefiting our patient population. The technology needed to acheive these goals is rapidly becoming a reality.

Dr. Firouz Daneshgari is certainly to be congratulated for developing this issue of the *Urologic Clinics of North America*, in which he has brought together individuals of varying expertise in this evolving field. The topics discussed represent a wide perspective, ranging from adults to children and from patients who are symptomatic of bladder dysfunction for causes that are not readily identifiable to those who have specific neurologic disorders.

On first look, one may question whether the topics in this issue have any value for the practicing urologist. How do they necessarily impact typical clinical activities? Upon closer examination, it becomes readily apparent that many of the topics are very pertinent. It also becomes apparent that as this technology improves, patients will be questioning and seeking these treatments, which with increasing experience will likely result in increased benefits.

Martin I. Resnick, MD
Lester Persky Professor and Chairman
Department of Urology
Case Western Reserve University
School of Medicine/University Hospitals
11100 Euclid Avenue
Cleveland, OH 44106, USA

E-mail address: mir@po.cwru.edu

ELSEVIER
SAUNDERS

Urol Clin N Am 32 (2005) xiii–xiv

UROLOGIC
CLINICS
of North America

Preface

Pelvic Neuromodulation

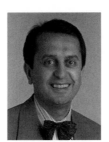

Firouz Daneshgari, MD
Guest Editor

In 1863, Giannuzzi stimulated the spinal cord in dogs and concluded that the hypogastric and pelvic nerves are involved in regulation of the bladder. What he set in motion for the next 150 years of testing in the field of neurouroloy is the concept that nerve stimulation can correct or control the function of pelvic organs. Although Giannuzzi might never have envisioned such methods of "neuromodulation" as stimulation of sacral, obturator, pudendal, or peripheral nerves or insertion of miniature devices or injection of neurotoxins into the bladder—these techniques have been tested and applied in laboratories and clinical settings throughout the world.

However, the recent success and subsequent regulatory approval of a sacral neuromodulation device has engergized the field and has created an historic surge in both clinical usage and the research activities related to pelvic neuromodulation. This surge in activities related to neuromodulation has been driven by a very human medical dilemma: the limited therapeutic options available to patients who suffer from pelvic organ diseases—and the pressing need to be more efficient and less invasive in our neuromodulatory approaches.

As in other areas in medicine, we're looking for those sparks of success that will lead to creative fires of expanding knowledge. But we also need to respect the well-established integrity of our field by being true to our surgeon-scientist tools as we

protect and explore the increasing territory of pelvic neuromodulation. This issue of the *Urologic Clinics of North America* seeks to spotlight our track record of integrity.

It has been a rare privilege for me to lead a group of international experts in producing this first-ever issue of the *Urologic Clinics of North America* dedicated to pelvic neuromodulation, a work that was created with several goals in mind. We wanted to provide the first comprehensive, reader-friendly guide on the topic for practitioners who deal with pelvic floor disorders. We also believe it is important to define what is currently the state-of-the-art in this field. Finally, we hoped to create an investigative platform that will allow us to peer wisely into the future of pelvic neuromodulation.

In this issue, we've tried to present you with a panoramic view of pelvic neuromodulation. The articles are organized so that readers with varying degrees of interest can find the information they require. We begin with past historical aspects and conclude with a glance to the future. In between, we offer technical expertise on how to conduct these procedures and detailed information on patient selection and troubleshooting. We travel to Canada and Europe to provide international clinical data, and we pose all the pertinent research questions on the clinically available modalities from sacral to peripheral to insertable devices and injectable agents. Additionally, this

0094-0143/05/$ - see front matter © 2005 Elsevier Inc. All rights reserved.
doi:10.1016/j.ucl.2004.11.003

urologic.theclinics.com

issue provides all the currently available clinical applications of neuromodulation for urinary incontinence, bladder dysfunction, fecal incontinence, and pediatric use.

I am indebted to the authors for their contributions to this comprehensive and updated publication on pelvic neuromodulation, and I applaud their success in completing these articles on a very tight timetable.

It is my sincere hope that this work will inspire additional enthusiasm in the field of neurourology, and that this enthusiasm will be directed toward addressing relevant research questions in pelvic neuromodulation. There is a danger here. Ignoring unexplored issues in this field will create an overhanging cloud that could dampen professional enthusiasm and ultimately limit the potential of this useful therapeutic modality.

So let's continue to fuel our fire of expanding knowledge. I'd like to dedicate this issue to the pioneers in our field who sparked us on this path and to the upcoming generation of surgeon-scientists in the area of pelvic medicine and reconstructive surgery who will furnish the light necessary to lead us to the next level of pelvic neuromodulation.

Firouz Daneshgari, MD
Director, Center for Female Pelvic Medicine &
Reconstructive Surgery
The Cleveland Clinic Foundation
Glickman Urological Institute
9500 Euclid Avenue A100
Cleveland, OH 44195, USA

E-mail address: daneshf@ccf.org

ELSEVIER
SAUNDERS

Urol Clin N Am 32 (2005) xv–xvi

UROLOGIC
CLINICS
of North America

Introduction

Neuromodulation: Past, Present, and Future

The concept of in vivo nerve stimulation to alter physiologic processes that cause symptoms originated in the nineteenth century. Advances in technology permitted this approach to bloom in the late twentieth century for the treatment of neuromuscular disorders, pain, and urologic conditions. Pioneering work by Tanagho, Brindley, and Schmidt led to clinical trials of implantable devices to treat genitourinary disorders including erectile dysfunction, urinary incontinence, interstitial cystitis, and urinary retention. Recently added to this list is use for fecal incontinence. However, clinical use often preceded a thorough understanding of the mechanisms whereby these devices improve such a wide array of conditions. Neuromodulation has expanded beyond the laboratory and academic centers to community practice. The adoption of these methods by community urologists reflects the frustration of patients and physicians with current behavioral and pharmacologic regimens for urge incontinence, pelvic pain, and retention. Indeed, patients often plead for anything that has the hope of relieving these very bothersome symptoms.

A more complete understanding of the sites, transmitters, and pathways regulating the genitourinary tract permits testable hypotheses regarding how stimulation of peripheral autonomic and somatic nerves—as well as areas within the central nervous system—improve conditions such as urge urinary incontinence. Complicating this understanding has been the realization that nerves change their function and sometimes signaling methods in response to disease, injury, and even repeated electrical stimulation. These alterations have been generically termed *neural plasticity*.

Simplistically, it has been thought that stimulation of sacral nerves leads to release of neurotransmitters that inhibit bladder function, a model used to explain efficacy of acupuncture. In addition, long-term changes as inferred from increased production of proto-oncogene products and neurotrophins has been postulated. However, the universal observation that discontinuation of nerve stimulation after years of functioning results in the immediate return of symptoms indicates this modality works acutely. Thus long-term plasticity triggered by stimulation may be unlikely. In clinical trials the finding that certain areas of the brain exhibit increased activity correlating with efficacy implies that supraspinal sites play an important role in addition to spinal sites.

Advances on two fronts will allow improvements in our ability to stimulate nerves and produce desirable effects on genitourinary function. First, more detailed neurophysiologic information is needed to design devices targeting plasticity in neural pathways. For example, if changes in Na/K channels in bladder afferents occur in response to inflammation, injury, or obstruction of the lower urinary tract and contribute to increased afferent activity, it may be possible to set parameters that reverse or improve the environment for nerve function. Knowledge of how magnetic and electrical fields alter cellular function is needed. Second, advances in technology, including nanotechnology, will allow miniaturization of devices and improved acceptance among clinicians and patients. It is possible that multimodal therapies that combine neuromodulation with neurotoxins or small-molecule drug therapies may be desirable in some conditions. For example, botulinum toxin A may be needed to transiently reduce neurotransmitter release, whereas subsequent nerve stimulation could prevent return of overactivity. It appears intuitively obvious that insights into pathophysiology and risk factors may identify those patients that are best served by neuromodulation.

Risk/benefit and cost/benefit ratios must be carefully weighed for patients undergoing implantation of neuromodulatory devices. Given the enthusiastic reports in the literature for devices

0094-0143/05/$ - see front matter © 2005 Elsevier Inc. All rights reserved.
doi:10.1016/j.ucl.2004.11.001

urologic.theclinics.com

such as InterStim (Medtronic) in patients failing behavioral and pharmacologic therapies, one wonders why this approach has not been more widely used. Data on durability and ideal candidates are now appearing from pioneering sites. Yet large-scale randomized studies—especially comparator studies with different modes of neuromodulation—are needed instead of relatively small numbers of patients from a large number of institutions. A national registry would clarify these issues.

Although the best patients for implantation are still debatable, and prescreening is often required, some individuals seem to fare poorly in the long term. These patients include those with chronic pain, complete lesions (in cord-injured patients), or neurologic disease. Such failures provide insight into the mechanisms that prevent neuromodulation from working in expected ways.

This issue of the *Urologic Clinics of North America* tackles some of these issues and reviews a growing world experience. It features a group of highly distinguished experts in the field who relate their experiences with this modality. The current enthusiasm is tempered by the realization that neuromodulation is not a panacea; therefore, further advances are needed before this approach has more widespread appeal.

William D. Steers, MD, FACS
Hovey Dabney Professor & Chair
Department of Urology
University of Virginia School of Medicine
Box 800422
Charlottesville, VA 22908, USA

ELSEVIER
SAUNDERS

Urol Clin N Am 32 (2005) 1–10

UROLOGIC
CLINICS
of North America

Neuromodulation in Voiding Dysfunction: A Historical Overview of Neurostimulation and its Application

Thomas Fandel, MD, Emil A. Tanagho, MD*

Department of Urology, University of California School of Medicine, San Francisco, CA 94143–0738, USA

The history of neuromodulation and neurostimulation has its beginnings in important discoveries in the fields of electricity and neurophysiology because humankind did not appreciate the associations among nerves, electricity, and muscle contraction until the middle of the eighteenth century. Furthermore, only natural electricity, as in the torpedo fish and static electricity, was known [1].

In antiquity, people believed that muscle contractions were the result of "animal spirits" in the brain, which were then conducted to the muscles via hollow nerves [2]. This theory persisted into the eighteenth century. Caldani in Bologna demonstrated in 1756 that electrical irritation of a nerve was a powerful stimulus that induced muscular convulsion [3]. In 1786, Galvani [4] produced muscle contraction by touching a nerve and its muscle with a combination of two different metals and concluded that electricity and "nerve fluid" were one and the same. He thought that this electricity was stored in the muscle fibers, however, and called this phenomenon "animal electricity." In 1792, Volta produced muscle contractions by touching both ends of different metals to the nerve only, and described the principle of current [5]. He reasoned that the electrical nerve fluid could be set in motion only by the metals' dissimilarity and dismissed the concept of animal electricity. Von Humboldt, who introduced the term "galvanism" for current [6], proved in 1797 that muscular

convulsions were the result of electricity in the animal itself. He achieved contractions in an experimental setting consisting of a muscle and the adjacent nerve looping back to it [7].

In 1811, Bell was the first to conduct experiments on the spinal nerve roots [8]. His anatomic studies showed that manipulation of the intradural anterior fasciculus led to muscle convulsions of the back, whereas cutting across the posterior fasciculus of nerves resulted in no contractions [9]. Bell drew the conclusion, however, that the anterior nerve roots, connected to the cerebrum, conduct sensory and motor impulses. In his concept, the posterior nerve roots were connected to the cerebellum and accounted for the vital functions. Magendie was the first to conduct a physiologic investigation of spinal nerve roots [8]. In radiculotomy studies on young puppies he found that cutting the posterior root extinguished sensation, although movement was still present [10], whereas cutting the anterior root abolished movement, but sensation was still present. He postulated that nerve roots consist of an anterior efferent motor portion and a posterior afferent sensory portion. It was not until 1833 that Hall [11] uncovered a distinct function of the spinal cord and medulla oblongata: that of reflex action. These first perceptions formed the basis for further examinations of organ innervation by the autonomic nervous system.

Knowledge of the neurologic associations among spinal marrow, nerves, and the urinary bladder arose after the middle of the nineteenth century. In 1863, Giannuzzi [12] stimulated the spinal cord in dogs and concluded that the hypogastric and pelvic nerves are involved in regulation of the bladder. In 1872, Budge [13] postulated two sets of nerves governing the

This work was supported in part by Deutsche Forschungsgemeinschaft No. FA 479/1-1.

* Corresponding author.

E-mail address: etanagho@urol.ucsf.edu (E.A. Tanagho).

bladder: one in the anterior roots of S1-S3 (motor); another in the hypogastric plexus (sensory). Sokownin reported that stimulation of the cut peripheral ends of the hypogastric nerves caused bladder contraction [described in 14]. Sherrington [15] gave a detailed account of the lumbosacral plexus in animal studies in 1892, concluding from stimulation of anterior roots that the nerve supply of the bladder in cats originates mainly in L3-L5 and S1-S3, and in monkeys from L2-L4 and S1-S3. On the basis of these observations, Langley and Anderson [14] succeeded in describing the sympathetic and parasympathetic effects on the bladder. They revealed the motor innervation of the detrusor muscle by selective rhizotomy of different fibers of the pelvic nerve (with electrical stimulation of the distal ends) and hypogastric nerve.

Budge [16] hypothesized a micturition center in the S2-S4 region in 1864. By 1900, Stewart [17] suggested a center of bladder evacuation in the lumbar spine. In 1958, Nathan and Smith [18] demonstrated the central neural pathways of the bladder in the spinal cord. The micturition center itself—as a complex of parasympathetic neural connections—lies in the intermediate gray areas located in the lateral column of S2-S4.

In 1820, Oersted discovered that a current-carrying wire had magnetic properties [19], describing the long-suspected connection between electricity and magnetism. Conversely, in 1833 Faraday concluded that a magnetic field could invoke current in a wire [20]. In his experiments he demonstrated that current changes in a primary circuit (and changing magnetic fields) caused a current in a secondary circuit. Faraday had discovered induced current.

The principle of the induction coil also had significance for electrostimulation because it laid the foundation for remote-controlled, completely implantable, neurostimulators. The stimulator devised by Light and Chaffee in 1934 [21] avoided the risk of infection from percutaneous leads by implanting a secondary coil underneath the skin. The primary coil was placed outside the body, using magnetic induction for energy transfer and modulation. Following the description of the electromagnetic wave by Hertz in 1892 and the discovery of high-frequency oscillations [22], it became possible to stimulate neural tissue by transmitting high-frequency alternating current inductively [23]. Glenn et al [24] used this principle when they developed an implantable receiver triggered by radiofrequency transmission for electrical stimulation.

The first attempt at electrical bladder stimulation may date back to 1878, when the Danish surgeon Saxtorph treated patients with urinary retention by intravesical stimulation [25], in which he inserted a special catheter with a metal electrode transurethrally. It was not until the 1940s, however, that further efforts were undertaken. The central question was: Which part of the neuromuscular pathway for micturition should be chosen to initiate voiding in urinary retention or to prevent voiding in incontinence? Numerous techniques were developed and may be classified according to the location of electrical stimulation as follows: transurethral bladder stimulation, direct detrusor stimulation, pelvic nerve stimulation, pelvic floor stimulation, spinal cord stimulation, and sacral root stimulation.

Transurethral bladder stimulation

Diseases of the spinal cord and plexuses inhibit the efferent impulses regulating depolarization processes at the periphery, so that receptors become unexcitable. Katona's group [26] began transurethral electrical stimulation in 1958 with a technique derived from Saxtorph. According to their hypothesis, stimulation of intramural bladder receptors in patients with incomplete central or peripheral nerve lesions may reactivate these receptors and recreate vegetative afferentation from the bladder to the central nervous system followed by enhancement of detrusor reflex. In 1975, they reported 420 patients treated with this method, of whom 314 achieved micturition control. In 1982, Madersbacher et al [27] presented a series of 30 patients treated in a similar manner, of whom 17 gained bladder control and 10 became dry.

Direct detrusor stimulation

In 1954, McGuire performed direct bladder stimulation in dogs to examine the optimal parameters required for detrusor contraction (described in [28]). He concluded that maximal muscle response was obtained by surge variation of either sine or rectangular wave forms with 15 V and a frequency of 15 to 60 Hz. The electrode material seemed not to influence the results; a wire coil or perforated plate (not exceeding 1–1.5 cm in diameter) appeared to be equally effective. McGuire realized that a single pair of electrodes did not effect a uniform spread of the stimulus, but multiple pairs gave a more uniform increase in intravesical pressure. These studies were continued by Boyce et al [28]. They found that two or more bipolar wire electrodes, consisting of two parallel wires, produced a more uniform response than a single lead in each of the same positions, generating multiple small electrical fields within the detrusor muscle. The same group used an induction coil for direct bladder stimulation in three paraplegic men with complete paralysis of the detrusor muscle. The wire electrodes were coiled and completely implanted into the bladder musculature. The results were unqualified failure in one, partial success in another, and a highly successful response in the third [28].

In 1962, Bradley et al [29] reported their experiments with an implantable stimulator in which radiofrequency transmission was used to trigger the receiver. Disk and tape electrodes were attached to the bladder wall in dogs. The first results were promising, achieving complete bladder evacuation in acute and chronic models over 13 months [30]. The results were not reproducible, however, in humans [31]. Detrusor contraction was induced on stimulation, but bladder evacuation occurred in only two patients, whereas in several patients current spread to the striated muscles was seen.

Several groups came forward in the early 1960s with experiments on direct detrusor stimulation in the bladder wall or the vicinity of the bladder. Tscholl et al [32] addressed electrode placement and type, which influenced the optimal current to empty the bladder (wire electrodes 15–25 V [33,34] or disk electrodes 10–45 V [29,35]). The high current densities necessary to achieve micturition (because of sluggish conduction across the smooth muscle) have been a major problem in these methods, resulting in tissue damage and stimulation of the pelvic floor.

New electrodes were developed to confine current to the bladder muscle and reduce current density. In 1968, Susset and Boctor [36] described their electrode, consisting of eight electrode disks. By implanting the disks in the upper half of the detrusor muscle in two circles of alternating polarities around the bladder, they achieved bladder contractions with 10 to 15 V without pelvic floor contractions. In this same report the authors summarized 20 cases of direct detrusor stimulation in humans from the literature. In 8 of 12 patients with upper motor neuron lesions, complete failure resulted, as it did in three of six patients with lower motor neuron lesions and in two unspecified cases. In 1969, Timm and Bradley [37] attached three

bipolar wire electrodes with small square tabs of alternating polarities to the bladder. They minimized current fields by applying electrical pulses sequentially. Tscholl et al [32] were able to show in 1971 that a further separation of electrode disks resulted in effectiveness with lower currents, and they developed an electrode derived from Susset and Boctor's, consisting of 20 small disks.

In 1966, Hald et al [38] demonstrated that the increase in urethral resistance is dependent on the voltage and frequency used for bladder stimulation. They introduced electrically induced sphincter fatigue for improved voiding with detrusor stimulation. Furthermore, they realized that intermittent short periods of stimulation prolonged the effect of sphincter fatigue.

In 1967, Habib [39] described the concept of trigger points for the urinary bladder (ie, areas that need only weak stimuli for efficient detrusor contraction). Stimulation of these points can successfully induce voiding without pain or contraction of adjoining muscles.

In 1978, Jonas and Hohenfellner [40] analyzed the efficacy of direct bladder stimulation in patients. Results were disappointing, because this procedure was successful in only 1 of 11 patients; seven patients developed reflex evacuation and the remaining three patients showed no function at all.

Advantages of this method are easy placement of electrodes, high specificity of target organ, and direct application in lower motor neuron lesions [41]. Disadvantages are occasional electrode malfunction from movement during voiding, production of fibrosis, erosion into the bladder, and the need for current densities above physiologic levels associated with stimulation of adjacent motor nerves.

Pelvic nerve stimulation

In 1940 and 1941, Dees [42] studied bladder contraction followed by activation of the pelvic nerves. For this purpose, he stimulated the hypogastric pelvic plexus on the lateral and anterior walls of the rectum with a bipolar electrode transrectally. In cats, he achieved vigorous contractions of the detrusor muscle along with simultaneous contraction of the urethral sphincter. This resulted in an intermittent escape of a few drops of fluid. Effective currents produced pain and contraction in the muscles of the hind legs. Although the human hypogastric plexus is farther from the perineum, contraction of the perineal muscles and penile erection occurred on stimulation. Pain became a limiting factor, and no bladder contractions resulted.

In 1957, Ingersoll et al [43] examined the effects of unilateral stimulation of pelvic nerves. They consistently found strong contractions on the stimulated side and varying results on the contralateral side. Burghele et al [44] presented their experience with radiofrequency-induced pelvic nerve stimulation in 1962. They obtained smooth sphincter contractions during voiding and attributed this phenomenon to current flow into the hypogastric nerves at the level of the pelvic plexus. Holmquist and Olin [45] elucidated the factors causing outflow resistance through the urethra during electrostimulation of pelvic nerves. They demonstrated that stimulation of intact pelvic nerves resulted in antidromic stimulation of the external sphincter via the pudendal nerves. Furthermore, engorgement of the erectile tissue constricted the perineal urethra. In 1968, Holmquist [46] presented the long-term results of stimulation of pelvic nerves in 25 dogs: one showed good bladder contractions over 2 years; in the others contraction gradually became weaker in response to a constant stimulus. He ascribed this phenomenon to the growth of connective tissue between the nerves and the electrodes.

Hald et al [47] in 1966 examined the influence of electrical stimulation on the integrity of pelvic nerves. Over the long-term, the pressure responses steadily declined and the electrical threshold increased. Histologic evaluation revealed a gradual deterioration in their dogs, with bulky roughened nerve trunks imbedded in dense scar tissue, increasing resistance to stimulation.

Pelvic nerves seem not to tolerate stimulation for long periods [41]. With this method, pudendal nerves are activated, resulting in augmented outflow resistance; pain is increased via the hypogastric nerves and the bladder nerves may be damaged permanently. Additionally, in humans the fibers of the parasympathetic nervous system innervating the bladder split early in their course through the pelvis, forming a plexus unsuitable for electrode application.

Pelvic floor stimulation

In 1963, Caldwell [48] reported his clinical experience with the first implantable pelvic floor stimulator. This device had been developed originally for fecal incontinence: the electrodes were inserted into the anal sphincter and the secondary coil of a radiofrequency transformer was implanted. In the same year, Caldwell et al [49] treated a patient with urinary incontinence with this method. After insertion of the electrodes into the external urethral sphincter, the patient gained complete continence at night and was able to void about every 4 hours during the day.

Several external stimulators were developed in the following years because the implanted device showed a high incidence of technical failure and electrode dislocation. Hopkinson and Lightwood [50] designed an anal plug stimulator for anal incontinence and in 1967 reported results for the treatment of urinary incontinence [51]. Alexander and Rowan [52] described a vaginal pessary stimulator in 1968. Although they achieved improvement in female patients with stress incontinence, success was short-lived [53].

Another approach for intravaginal stimulation of pelvic floor muscles was presented by Erlandson et al [54] in 1977. They introduced a cylindrical vaginal plug, to which electrodes were attached. Experiments in cats demonstrated that intravaginal stimulation caused urethral closure and simultaneous bladder inhibition. These two effects were optimal, however, at different stimulation parameters. Fall et al [55] showed that intravaginal stimulation activated several neuronal pathways. Direct stimulation of pudendal nerve efferents to the striated paraurethral and pelvic floor muscles caused urethral closure. Bladder inhibition was the result of two spinal reflex mechanisms: stimulation of the pudendal nerve afferents resulted in reflexogenic activation of hypogastric efferents and central inhibition of the pelvic efferents [56]. In another account, Fall et al [57] reported long-term intravaginal stimulation in patients with urge and stress incontinence: results were successful in seven of nine patients with pure stress incontinence and in 15 patients with detrusor instability or mixed incontinence.

In 1983, McGuire et al [58] used transcutaneous stimulation of the common peroneal or posterior tibial nerve for inhibition of detrusor activity. This method seemed to have less current loss than with the anal plug electrode. Although simple, it never found widespread acceptance.

Spinal cord stimulation

In the late 1960s, Nashold et al [59] began experiments with spinal cord stimulation. By activating the micturition center, they attempted to achieve greater coordination. The group compared the effectiveness of stimulating the dorsal surface of the spinal marrow with depth stimulation in acute and chronic studies [60]. Surface stimulation at S2 resulted in the highest bladder pressure, although no voiding occurred because of the absence of external sphincter relaxation. Bladder emptying was achieved only by insertion of bipolar electrodes into the sacral intermediolateral portion of the central gray matter at S1-S2 (the micturition center). They concluded that successful stimulation was dependent on location and frequency and voltage.

Nashold et al [61] transferred the experience gained to humans and in 1972 reported the first four patients with stimulator implants. In a subsequent review after the first 10 years, they reported a total of 27 neuroprosthetic implants worldwide and set the overall success rate at 55.6% [62]. A good postoperative result was defined as voiding large amounts of urine with stimulation and exhibiting low urinary residual and reduced infection. Their own clinical series included 14 patients (seven male, seven female); 10 patients (four male, six female) experienced a good result with conus stimulation from 3 to 8 years [63]. Of this group, two male patients needed either a bladder neck resection or a partial sphincterotomy.

Jonas et al [64] examined the parameters for most effective stimulation of the spinal cord in 1975. They compared different types of electrodes, different stimulation parameters (voltage, frequency, and optimal level), and results of spinal stimulation before and after acute transection above the micturition center in dogs. They concluded that results did not depend on electrode type: the wraparound surface electrode with the most extended current spread provoked the same results as the coaxial electrode with the least current spread. This observation led them to conjecture that it may be impossible to isolate the detrusor center from a sphincteric center for stimulation. Optimal stimulation parameters were 2 to 5 V and 10 to 15 Hz for 1 millisecond. The best level of stimulation could not be determined because the sphincteric response was elicited from a large area exceeding about one quarter of a level both above and below the area of detrusor response. No voiding could be achieved in the uninjured dog because of simultaneous contraction of the detrusor and sphincteric muscles. After spinal cord transection, however, a spurt of urine occurred at the end of each stimulus and they called this phenomenon "poststimulus voiding."

Jonas and Tanagho [65] demonstrated that the muscle response of the bladder after spinal cord transection rose and dropped more slowly than that of the urethral sphincter. At the end of the stimulus there was a short time when bladder pressure exceeded sphincteric pressure (the spurt of urine). Repetitive stimuli resulted in complete bladder evacuation. In the same year Jonas et al [66] compared the efficiency of micturition induced by spinal cord stimulation with direct bladder stimulation. They concluded that the net effective voiding pressure was lower and bladder evacuation less after stimulation of the spinal cord; direct bladder stimulation seemed to be a better and more specific tool for voiding.

Thüroff et al [67] performed retrograde neurotracer studies to distinguish the micturition center from the sphincteric center in the spinal cord. They succeeded in separating the parasympathetic nucleus from the somatic nucleus and demonstrated that most parasympathetic neurons were located in the intermediolateral and intermediomedial cell column of the gray region of S2. In contrast, the somatic neurons were mainly confined to Onuf's nucleus in S1 and S2. Although no overlap was evident on horizontal sections, the parasympathetic nucleus could be shown within the area of the pudendal nucleus in the vertical dimension.

These findings demonstrate that stimulation of the micturition center is feasible and results in voiding, but simultaneous activation of the sphincter interferes profoundly.

Sacral root stimulation

In 1972, Brindley [68] presented an electrode array for chronic electrical connection to spinal roots. After laminectomy and opening of the dura mater, split strands of anterior roots were inserted into slots of the implant. On stimulation of the first and second sacral ventral root in baboons, he achieved emptying of the bladder or closure of the urethra [69]. This phenomenon is caused by the fact that somatic nerve fibers are larger than the parasympathetic fibers and more electrically sensitive. Weak electrical stimuli resulted in activation only of the striated closure muscles [70]. Using continuous stimulation at 20 Hz with a voltage maximal for somatic nerve fibers but subliminal for bladder contraction, he obtained urethral closure for 3 minutes. Strong electrical stimuli activated both the detrusor muscle of the bladder and the striated sphincter muscles.

Because smooth muscle relaxes much more slowly than striated muscle, Brindley achieved micturition by delivering bursts for 1 second (40 V, 0.1 millisecond, 50 Hz) with stimulation:rest ratio of 2:1. The bladder contracted smoothly, whereas the striated muscles relaxed in the intervals, and female baboons consistently emptied the bladder successfully. From 1976, Brindley et al [71] began implanting sacral anterior root stimulators in paraplegic patients with incontinence and in 1986 they presented their experience with the first 50 cases. Of the 49 patients alive, 30 were completely continent and 5 were continent at night; 43 patients regularly used their implants for micturition and 26 of 38 male patients were able to produce penile erection under stimulation. In 1986, Sauerwein [72] combined sacral anterior root stimulation with sacral deafferentation in patients with spinal cord lesions to overcome reflex urinary incontinence. Rhizotomy of the posterior roots of S2 to S5 in 45 patients resulted in abolition of spasticity in 93% and secure continence in 91%.

Tanagho and coworkers used the canine model for sacral root stimulation because the anatomy of the sacral nerves is similar to that in humans. They stimulated the extradural intraspinal segment to maintain the cerebrospinal fluid chamber intact. In 1977, Heine et al [73] identified the sacral root producing maximal detrusor contraction and minimal outflow resistance. S2 consistently produced the strongest bladder contractions associated with significant sphincteric response. In contrast, S1 produced strong sphincteric contraction but little bladder response. Schmidt et al [74] selectively stimulated different parts of S2, but obtained comparable results from both dorsal and ventral roots. They attributed this effect to central reflex pathways. Furthermore, stimulation of the intact root or the dorsal component alone was least effective, whereas stimulation of the anterior component resulted in good voiding with low residual urine volume. They concluded that unwanted sphincter contraction reflexes via the spinal cord might be significantly diminished by performing a posterior rhizotomy to achieve maximal response from the detrusor. Stimulation of the ventral root of S2 caused detrusor contraction and sphincteric response because of the presence of both parasympathetic and somatic fibers. Schmidt et al [75] investigated the effect of selective division of the somatic fibers or complete section of the pudendal nerve. After somatic neurotomy, the response to

stimulation of the entire nerve was not significantly different. Only stimulation of the dorsal peripheral nerve end after dorsal rhizotomy yielded diminished sphincteric activity. Stimulation of the central nerve end resulted in efficient sphincter reflex contraction that was eliminated only through subsequent successive division of all remaining sacral nerves. Most of the sphincteric response was lost with division of S1 and S2 bilaterally. The authors reasoned that the reflex pathways available for sphincteric control were far more numerous or far more efficient than those for micturition. Posterior rhizotomy seemed to be mandatory because somatic stimuli could otherwise be generously integrated within the spinal cord. Selective division of somatic fibers or complete section of the pudendal nerve showed an equal effect. In the final model they separated the dorsal fibers, cut the dorsal component, stimulated the ventral component, and performed selective neurotomy of the stimulated root while sparing all other somatic fibers carried along other sacral roots to maintain activity of the pudendal nerve.

In 1982, Tanagho and Schmidt [76] presented the first results of sacral root stimulation in paraplegic dogs. The experience from this study resulted in the design of a spiral electrode to minimize nerve damage. Fixation of the lead wire directly to the sacral lamina prevented tension on the electrode. With this electrode in chronic experiments with spinal cord injured dogs, persistently good voiding was obtained with good bladder contraction and almost no sphincteric response [77]. Thüroff et al [78] performed several chronic studies in spinal cord injured dogs after dorsal rhizotomy and ganglionectomy. To obtain micturition by stimulating S2, they turned the different fatigue patterns in smooth and striated muscles to account. The striated sphincter, which is composed of slow- and fast-twitch fibers, is easily fatigable because of the proportion of fast-twitch fibers. Fatiguing the fast-twitch fibers, which account for the dyssynergic urethral resistance, leaves only the very fatigue-resistant smooth and striated slow-twitch activity. This remaining urethral resistance was easy to overcome and did not prevent complete bladder evacuation, which they achieved with high-frequency (200 Hz), low-voltage stimulation followed by high-voltage stimulation. In a different account, Thüroff et al [79] evaluated the optimal stimulation parameters to induce and maintain urethral closure. Continuous low-voltage stimulation of S2 induced fatigue of the contracted external sphincter. Phasic stimulation with bursts of 30 to 60 milliseconds and a stimulation:rest ratio of 1:2, however, resulted in unfused sphincteric tetany and a sufficient sphincteric closure pressure over 1 hour of stimulation. In 1983, they reported their experience with chronic extradural stimulation of sacral roots: as long as 8 months and a cumulative time of 100 to 150 hours [80]. They concluded that long-term stimulation did not induce neural impairment because threshold parameters for stimulation remained exactly the same over the period. Histologic evaluation revealed preservation of axonal integrity in the ventral roots, whereas the severed dorsal root fibers showed degeneration.

On the basis of these results, Tanagho [81] started first human clinical trials in 1982. Stimulation of sacral root S3 generally induced detrusor and sphincteric action. S2 stimulation typically produced inward rotation of the leg, whereas S4 stimulation generally resulted in contraction of the levator ani and frequently in a bladder response [82]. After several variations, Tanagho performed electrode implantation on the ventral root of S3 or S4 combined with extensive dorsal rhizotomy and selective peripheral neurotomy. It was concluded that this model was the most successful combination to achieve continence and promote bladder evacuation. In 1990, Tanagho [83] reported on the first 35 patients suffering from neuropathic voiding dysfunction caused by suprasegmental spinal cord lesions: of 25 patients available for follow-up, 60% experienced restored reservoir function and continence and complete bladder evacuation.

In neuroanatomic studies, Hohenfellner et al [84] tried to attenuate the risk of detrusor-sphincter dyssynergia after stimulation of the ventral sacral roots. They determined that dorsal sacral rhizotomy could be done more extensively if performed intradurally rather than extradurally. They also revealed that the ventral root could be subdivided into three to five rootlets from their point of origin in the spinal cord to their exit from the dural sac. Probst et al [85] demonstrated that the rootlets maintain their number and identity throughout the entire intradural course. This raised the possibility of identifying rootlets carrying fibers to the urethral sphincter predominantly and severing them selectively. Nevertheless, Hohenfellner et al [84] recommended extradural implantation of the electrodes to avoid the risk of accidental damage to the sacral anterior root, cerebrospinal fluid leakage, or myelomeningitis.

Parallel to the progress in neurostimulation, another development took place. Tanagho and Schmidt [77] observed that sphincteric contractions suppressed detrusor activity. Furthermore, pudendal nerve blockade improved bladder capacity [86]. They concluded, in accordance with Fall et al [55,56], that a reflex inhibitory mechanism exists between pelvic floor and detrusor activities. Excluding mechanical obstruction, Tanagho et al [77] classified the remaining voiding dysfunctions as related to the urinary bladder or the pelvic floor. To the latter group they ascribed severe urge and frequency caused by sphincteric instability and pelvic pain because of constant pelvic floor hyperactivity [87]. In response to the question of whether diminished urethral sphincter and pelvic floor instability may stabilize the entire micturition reflex mechanism, Tanagho [88] presented the concept of neuromodulation. Activation of the external sphincter by sacral root stimulation inhibited detrusor activity as a normal reflex phenomenon and minimized detrusor instability. The mechanism of action, which requires intact sensory pathways, is not completely understood. Because the parameters are too low to activate the autonomic component of the sacral root, stimulation primarily affects the somatic component in both the afferent sensory fibers and efferent motor fibers. Intraspinal connections between the pudendal and parasympathetic nuclei in the sacral segment are likely responsible for the modulation of the voiding reflex and detrusor activity.

In 1988, Schmidt [89] described the three stages of electrode placement. First, a needle was placed for test stimulation into the sacral foramina near the sacral roots. If the sacral nerve roots showed functional integrity and patients otherwise qualified for neuromodulation, the needle was replaced by a temporary wire for percutaneous stimulation. If the patient experienced an improvement in symptoms of urinary incontinence of over 50%, a permanent neural prosthesis was implanted. The electrode was inserted unilaterally either at the S3 foraminal level or at the level of the pudendal nerves.

A neuroprosthesis was first used for treatment of pelvic pain [90], and discomfort improved over 50% in 49% of patients. In 1990, Tanagho [91] presented the results of neurostimulation for incontinence. About 70% of 31 patients with urge incontinence obtained subjective improvement of 50% or more, as did 40% of 25 patients with postprostatectomy incontinence. Two years later,

Tanagho [92] published the results of neuromodulation in 27 children: five of seven children with meningomyelocele gained continence, as did four of six patients with voiding dysfunction and one of two patients with neonatal hypoxia.

In 1998, Shaker and Hassouna [93] evaluated the efficacy and safety of sacral root neuromodulation. Twenty patients with idiopathic nonobstructive chronic urinary retention gained at least 50% improvement in voided and postvoid residual volume on percutaneous nerve evaluation. After permanent implantation of the neurostimulator, patients significantly improved in voided volume and pelvic pain, and results tended to persist over the long term. They concluded that, for nonobstructive urinary retention, sacral root neuromodulation is an appealing, efficacious treatment. Implantation is relatively simple and carries a low complication rate.

References

[1] McNeal DR. 2000 years of electrical stimulation. In: Hambrecht FT, Reswick JB, editors. Functional electrical stimulation: applications in neural prostheses. Biomedical engineering and instrumentation series, vol. 3. New York: Marcel Dekker; 1977. p. 3–12.

[2] Rowbottom M, Susskind C. The discovery of a new form of electricity. In: Electricity and medicine: history of their interaction. San Francisco: San Francisco Press; 1984. p. 31.

[3] Pupilli GC. Introduction. In: Commentary on the effect of electricity on muscular motion; a translation of Luigi Galvani's De viribus electricitatis in motu musculari commentarius. Cambridge (MA): E. Licht; 1953. p. xi.

[4] Galvani L. Part III. The effects of animal electricity on muscular motion. In: Commentary on the effect of electricity on muscular motion; a translation of Luigi Galvani's De viribus electricitatis in motu musculari commentarius. Cambridge (MA): E. Licht; 1953. p. 40–59.

[5] Meyer M. Historischer Ueberblick über die Anwendung der Electricität in der Medicin. In: Die Electricität in ihrer Anwendung auf practische Medicin. 3rd edition. Berlin: A. Hirschwald; 1868. p. 3.

[6] Licht S. History of electrotherapy. In: Licht S, editor. Therapeutic electricity and ultraviolet radiation. 2nd edition. Physical medicine library, vol. 4. New Haven: E. Licht; 1967. p. 24.

[7] Von Humboldt FA. Zweiter Abschnitt. In: Versuche über die gereizte Muskel- und Nervenfaser. Posen: Decker und Compagnie and Berlin: HA. Rottman; 1797. p. 28–40.

[8] Cranefield PF. Bibliography. In: The way in and the way out: François Magendie, Charles Bell and the roots of the spinal nerves. Mount Kisco (NY): Futura Publishing Company; 1974. p. 11, 30.

[9] Bell C. Idea of a new anatomy of the brain; submitted for the observations of his friends. Printed in 1811 by Strahan and Preston, London; not published, but privately circulated. p. 1–36. Reprinted in: Cranefield PF, editor. The way in and the way out: François Magendie, Charles Bell and the roots of the spinal nerves. Mount Kisco (NY): Futura Publishing Company; 1974.

[10] Magendie F. Expériences sur les fonctions des racines des nerfs rachidiens. Journal de Physiologie Expérimentale et Pathologique 1822;2:276–9 (transl. Alexander CA). In: Flourens P, editor. Memoir of Magendie. 1858. p. 107–8. Reprinted in: Cranefield PF, editor. The way in and the way out. François Magendie, Charles Bell and the roots of the spinal nerves. Mount Kisco (NY): Futura Publishing Company; 1974.

[11] Hall M. On the reflex function of the medulla oblongata and medulla spinalis. Phil Trans 1833;123: 635–65.

[12] Giannuzzi J. Recherches physiologiques sur les nerfs moteurs de la vessie. Journal de la Physiologie de l'Homme et des Animaux 1863;6:22–9.

[13] Budge J. Zur physiologie des blasenschliessmuskels. Archiv für die gesammte Physiologie des Menschen und der Thiere 1872;6:306–11.

[14] Langley JN, Anderson HK. The innervation of the pelvic and adjoining viscera. Part II. The bladder. J Physiol 1895;19:71–84.

[15] Sherrington CS. Notes on the arrangement of some motor fibres in the lumbo-sacral plexus. Section III. Motor roots to muscles other than those of the limb. Of the urinary bladder. J Physiol 1892;13:676–83.

[16] Budge J. Ueber den Einfluss des Nervensystems auf die Bewegung der Blase. Z Rationelle Medicin 1864; 21:1–16.

[17] Stewart CC. Mammalian smooth muscle: the cat's bladder. Am J Physiol 1900;4:185–208.

[18] Nathan PW, Smith MC. The centrifugal pathway for micturition within the spinal cord. J Neurol Neurosurg Psychiatry 1958;21:177–89.

[19] Dibner B. Discovery of electromagnetism. In: Oersted and the discovery of electromagnetism. Norwalk (CT): Burndy Library; 1961. p. 16–21.

[20] Rowbottom M, Susskind C. Electromagnetism, electrodynamics, and first medical applications of varying currents. In: Electricity and medicine: history of their interaction. San Francisco: San Francisco Press; 1984. p. 56–7.

[21] Light RU, Chaffee EL. Electrical excitation of the nervous system. Introducing a new principle: remote control. Preliminary report. Science 1934;79: 299–300.

[22] Rowbottom M, Susskind C. D'Arsonval and high-frequency currents: the beginnings of diathermy. In: Electricity and medicine: history of their inter-

action. San Francisco: San Francisco Press; 1984. p. 128–9.

[23] Newman H, Fender F, Saunders W. High frequency transmission of stimulating impulses. Surgery 1937; 2:359–62.

[24] Glenn WW, Hageman JH, Mauro A, et al. Electrical stimulation of excitable tissue by radio-frequency transmission. Ann Surg 1964;160:338–50.

[25] Madersbacher H. Konservative Therapie der neurogenen Blasendysfunktion. Urologe A 1999;38:24–9.

[26] Katona F. Stages of vegetative afferentation in reorganization of bladder control during intravesical electrotherapy. Urol Int 1975;30:192–203.

[27] Madersbacher H, Pauer W, Reiner E, et al. Rehabilitation of micturition in patients with incomplete spinal cord lesions by transurethral electrostimulation of the bladder. Eur Urol 1982;8:111–6.

[28] Boyce WH, Lathem JE, Hunt LD. Research related to the development of an artificial electrical stimulator for the paralyzed human bladder: a review. J Urol 1964;91:41–51.

[29] Bradley WE, Wittmers LE, Chou SN, et al. Use of a radio transmitter receiver unit for the treatment of neurogenic bladder: a preliminary report. J Neurosurg 1962;19:782–6.

[30] Bradley WE, Wittmers LE, Chou SN. An experimental study of the treatment of the neurogenic bladder. J Urol 1963;90:575–82.

[31] Bradley WE, Chou SN, French LA. Further experience with the radio transmitter receiver unit for the neurogenic bladder. J Neurosurg 1963;20: 953–60.

[32] Tscholl R, Schreiter F, Jonas U. Direkte Stimulation des Detrusors mit einer simulierten Netzelektrode und transvasale Stimulation mit bipolaren Elektroden am Hund. Urologe A 1971;10:246–8.

[33] Kantrowitz A. Development of an implantable, externally controlled stimulator for the treatment of chronic cord bladder in paraplegic patients: report of three cases. Arch Phys Med Rehabil 1965;46: 76–8.

[34] Scott FB, Quesada EM, Cardus D, et al. Electronic bladder stimulation: dog and human experiments. Invest Urol 1965;3:231–43.

[35] Hageman J, Flanigan S, Harvard BM, et al. Electromicturition by radiofrequency stimulation. Surg Gynecol Obstet 1966;123:807–11.

[36] Susset JG, Boctor ZN. Implantable electrical vesical stimulator: clinical experience. J Urol 1967;98: 673–8.

[37] Timm GW, Bradley WE. Electrostimulation of the urinary detrusor to effect contraction and evacuation. Invest Urol 1969;6:562–8.

[38] Hald T, Freed PS, Agrawal G, et al. Urethral resistance during electrical stimulation. Invest Urol 1966;4:247–56.

[39] Habib HN. Experience and recent contributions in sacral nerve stimulation for voiding in both human and animal. Br J Urol 1967;39:73–83.

[40] Jonas U, Hohenfellner R. Late results of bladder stimulation in 11 patients: followup to 4 years. J Urol 1978;120:565–8.

[41] Tanagho EA. Induced micturition via intraspinal sacral root stimulation: clinical implications. In: Hambrecht FT, Reswick JB, editors. Functional electrical stimulation: applications in neural prostheses. Biomedical engineering and instrumentation series, vol. 3. New York: Marcel Dekker; 1977. p. 157–71.

[42] Dees JE. Contraction of the urinary bladder produced by electric stimulation: preliminary report. Invest Urol 1965;2:539–47.

[43] Ingersoll EH, Jones LL, Hegre ES. Effect on urinary bladder of unilateral stimulation of pelvic nerves in the dog. Am J Physiol 1957;189:167–72.

[44] Burghele T, Ichim V, Demetrescu M. Experimental study on emptying of the cord bladder. Transcutaneous stimulation of pelvic nerves by electromagnetic induction apparatus [paper 9]. In: Digest of the 1962 15th Annual Conference on Engineering in Medicine and Biology. Chicago: 1962. p. 58.

[45] Holmquist B, Olin T. Electromicturition in male dogs at pelvic nerve stimulation: an urethrocystographic study. Scand J Urol Nephrol 1968;2:115–27.

[46] Holmquist B. Electromicturition by pelvic nerve stimulation in dogs. Scand J Urol Nephrol Suppl 1968;2:1–27.

[47] Hald T, Agrawal G, Kantrowitz A. Studies in stimulation of the bladder and its motor nerves. Surgery 1966;60:848–56.

[48] Caldwell KP. The electrical control of sphincter incompetence. Lancet 1963;2:174–5.

[49] Caldwell KP, Flack FC, Broad AF. Urinary incontinence following spinal injury treated by electronic implant. Lancet 1965;1:846–7.

[50] Hopkinson BR, Lightwood R. Electrical treatment of anal incontinence. Lancet 1966;1:297–8.

[51] Hopkinson BR, Lightwood R. Electrical treatment of incontinence. Br J Surg 1967;54:802–5.

[52] Alexander S, Rowan D. An electric pessary for stress incontinence. Lancet 1968;1:728.

[53] Alexander S, Rowan D. Electrical control of urinary incontinence: a clinical appraisal. Br J Surg 1970;57: 766–8.

[54] Erlandson BE, Fall M, Carlsson CA. The effect of intravaginal electrical stimulation on the feline urethra and urinary bladder: electrical parameters. Scand J Urol Nephrol Suppl 1977;44:5–18.

[55] Fall M, Erlandson BE, Carlsson CA, et al. The effect of intravanginal electrical stimulation on the feline urethra and urinary bladder: neuronal mechanisms. Scand J Urol Nephrol Suppl 1977;44:19–30.

[56] Fall M. Electrical pelvic floor stimulation for the control of detrusor instability. Neurourol Urodyn 1985;4:329–35.

[57] Fall M, Erlandson BE, Nilson AE, et al. Long-term intravaginal electrical stimulation in urge and stress incontinence. Scand J Urol Nephrol Suppl 1977;44: 55–63.

[58] McGuire EJ, Zhang SC, Horwinski ER, et al. Treatment of motor and sensory detrusor instability by electrical stimulation. J Urol 1983;129:78–9.

[59] Nashold BS Jr, Friedman H, Boyarsky S. Electrical activation of micturition by spinal cord stimulation. J Surg Res 1971;11:144–7.

[60] Friedman H, Nashold BS Jr, Senechal P. Spinal cord stimulation and bladder function in normal and paraplegic animals. J Neurosurg 1972;36: 430–7.

[61] Nashold BS Jr, Friedman H, Glenn JF, et al. Electromicturition in paraplegia: implantation of a spinal neuroprosthesis. Arch Surg 1972;104:195–202.

[62] Nashold BS, Friedman H, Grimes J. Electrical stimulation of the conus medullaris to control bladder emptying in paraplegia: a ten-year review. Appl Neurophysiol 1982;45:40–3.

[63] Nashold BS Jr, Friedman H, Grimes J. Electrical stimulation of the conus medullaris to control the bladder in the paraplegic patient: a 10-year review. Appl Neurophysiol 1981;44:225–32.

[64] Jonas U, Heine JP, Tanagho EA. Studies on the feasibility of urinary bladder evacuation by direct spinal cord stimulation. I. Parameters of most effective stimulation. Invest Urol 1975;13:142–50.

[65] Jonas U, Tanagho EA. Studies on the feasibility of urinary bladder evacuation by direct spinal cord stimulation. II. Poststimulus voiding: a way to overcome outflow resistance. Invest Urol 1975;13:151–3.

[66] Jonas U, Jones LW, Tanagho EA. Spinal cord stimulation versus detrusor stimulation: a comparative study in six "acute" dogs. Invest Urol 1975;13: 171–4.

[67] Thüroff JW, Bazeed MA, Schmidt RA, et al. Regional topography of spinal cord neurons innervating pelvic floor muscles and bladder neck in the dog: a study by combined horseradish peroxidase histochemistry and autoradiography. Urol Int 1982;37:110–20.

[68] Brindley GS. Electrode-arrays for making long-lasting electrical connexion to spinal roots. J Physiol 1972;222:135P–6P.

[69] Brindley GS. Emptying the bladder by stimulating sacral ventral roots. J Physiol 1974;237:15P–6P.

[70] Brindley GS. An implant to empty the bladder or close the urethra. J Neurol Neurosurg Psychiatry 1977;40:358–69.

[71] Brindley GS, Polkey CE, Rushton DN, et al. Sacral anterior root stimulators for bladder control in paraplegia: the first 50 cases. J Neurol Neurosurg Psychiatry 1986;49:1104–14.

[72] Sauerwein D. Die operative Behandlung der spastischen Blasenlähmung bei Querschnittlähmung. Sakrale Deafferentation (SDAF) mit der Implantation eines sakralen Vorderwurzelstimulators (SARS). Urologe A 1990;29:196–203.

[73] Heine JP, Schmidt RA, Tanagho EA. Intraspinal sacral root stimulation for controlled micturition. Invest Urol 1977;15:78–82.

[74] Schmidt RA, Bruschini H, Tanagho EA. Urinary bladder and sphincter responses to stimulation of dorsal and ventral sacral roots. Invest Urol 1979; 16:300–4.

[75] Schmidt RA, Bruschini H, Tanagho EA. Sacral root stimulation in controlled micturition: peripheral somatic neurotomy and stimulated voiding. Invest Urol 1979;17:130–4.

[76] Tanagho EA, Schmidt RA. Bladder pacemaker: scientific basis and clinical future. Urology 1982;20: 614–9.

[77] Tanagho EA, Schmidt RA. Electrical stimulation in the clinical management of the neurogenic bladder. J Urol 1988;140:1331–9.

[78] Thüroff JW, Bazeed MA, Schmidt RA, et al. Functional pattern of sacral root stimulation in dogs. I. Micturition. J Urol 1982;127:1031–3.

[79] Thüroff JW, Bazeed MA, Schmidt RA, et al. Functional pattern of sacral root stimulation in dogs. II. Urethral closure. J Urol 1982;127:1034–8.

[80] Thüroff JW, Schmidt RA, Bazeed MA, et al. Chronic stimulation of the sacral roots in dogs. Eur Urol 1983;9:102–8.

[81] Tanagho EA. Neural stimulation for bladder control. Semin Neurol 1988;8:170–3.

[82] Tanagho EA, Schmidt RA, Orvis BR. Neural stimulation for control of voiding dysfunction: a preliminary report in 22 patients with serious neuropathic voiding disorders. J Urol 1989;142(2 Pt 1):340–5.

[83] Tanagho EA. Prinzipien und Indikationen der Elektrostimulation der Harnblase. Urologe A 1990;29: 185–90.

[84] Hohenfellner M, Paick JS, Trigo-Rocha F, et al. Site of deafferentation and electrode placement for bladder stimulation: clinical implications. J Urol 1992; 147:1665–70.

[85] Probst M, Piechota HJ, Hohenfellner M, et al. Neurostimulation for bladder evacuation: is sacral root stimulation a substitute for microstimulation? Br J Urol 1997;79:554–66.

[86] Schmidt RA. Technique of pudendal nerve localization for block or stimulation. J Urol 1989;142: 1528–31.

[87] Baskin LS, Tanagho EA. Pelvic pain without pelvic organs. J Urol 1992;147:683–6.

[88] Tanagho EA. Concepts of neuromodulation. Neurourol Urodyn 1993;12:487–8.

[89] Schmidt RA. Application of neurostimulation in urology. Neurourol Urodyn 1988;7:585–92.

[90] Schmidt RA. Treatment of pelvic pain with neuroprosthesis [abstract 458]. J Urol 1988;139:277A.

[91] Tanagho EA. Electrical stimulation. J Am Geriatr Soc 1990;38:352–5.

[92] Tanagho EA. Neuromodulation in the management of voiding dysfunction in children. J Urol 1992;148(2 Pt 2):655–7.

[93] Shaker HS, Hassouna M. Sacral root neuromodulation in idiopathic nonobstructive chronic urinary retention. J Urol 1998;159:1476–8.

ELSEVIER
SAUNDERS

Urol Clin N Am 32 (2005) 11–18

UROLOGIC
CLINICS
of North America

How Sacral Nerve Stimulation Neuromodulation Works

Wendy W. Leng, MD*, Michael B. Chancellor, MD

Department of Urology, University of Pittsburgh School of Medicine, 3471 Fifth Avenue, Suite #700, Pittsburgh, PA 15213, USA

The refractory overactive bladder represents one of the most challenging problems in urology. Current treatments for patients who have refractory overactive bladder or patients who cannot tolerate antimuscarinic pharmacotherapy are limited. For example, augmentation enterocystoplasty traditionally has been offered as a last resort in such situations. Intestinal augmentation using bowel, however, is a major operation with significant potential short-term and long-term complications. Even without complications, most patients are dismayed by the need for lifelong intermittent bladder catheterization after such reconstructive bladder surgery. Many patients refuse such therapies because the treatment may prove more troublesome than the disease [1].

Functional electrical stimulation is a nonsurgical modality that has proved effective for the condition of urge incontinence. Stimulation techniques have used surface electrodes, anal and vaginal plug electrodes [2–4], and dorsal penile nerve electrodes [5,6]. The theory underlying the mechanism of action of sacral nerve stimulation (SNS) is similar. Sacral neuromodulation, however, seems to offer the advantage of more durable, consistent control of lower urinary tract dysfunction. As a minimally invasive urologic procedure, it also has demonstrated long-term efficacy and safety. Furthermore, in addition to the treatment of refractory urge incontinence, sacral neuromodulation has been used to treat voiding dysfunction and idiopathic urinary retention.

This article discusses how SNS can treat the seemingly disparate spectrum of lower urinary tract dysfunctions—urinary urge incontinence, dysfunctional voiding, and idiopathic urinary retention [7–10]. The implantable system (Medtronic, Minneapolis, Minnesota) is comprised of a neurostimulator, an extension cable, and a lead with quadripolar electrodes. The electrode is implanted in one of the sacral foramen, most commonly the S3 foramen. The pulse generator later is implanted permanently in a subcutaneous pocket of the superior buttock. Subsequent adjustments of the stimulator impulse settings can be accomplished easily and noninvasively with an electronic programming device [11–14].

This article first discusses the pertinent neuroanatomy and neurophysiology relating to SNS. Understanding the fundamental blueprint of the central nervous system controls of micturition are essential to appreciating how SNS can treat a wide range of lower urinary tract dysfunctions.

Micturition reflexes

Normal micturition depends on neural pathways in the central nervous system. These pathways perform three major functions: amplification, coordination, and timing [16]. The nervous system control of the lower urinary tract must be able to amplify weak smooth muscle activity to provide sustained increases of intravesical pressures sufficient to empty the bladder. The bladder and urethral sphincter function must be coordinated to allow the sphincter to open during micturition but to remain closed at all other times. Timing reflects the volitional control of voiding that occurs with toilet training in human

Supported by National Institutes of Health grant 1K23 DK 62726-01/NIDDK.

* Corresponding author.
E-mail address: lengww@upmc.edu (W.W. Leng).

development. It also affords us the ability to initiate voiding over a wide range of bladder volumes (Fig. 1). In this regard, the bladder is a unique visceral organ that exhibits predominately voluntary rather than involuntary (autonomic) neural regulation. Several important reflex mechanisms contribute to the storage and elimination of urine and modulate the voluntary control of micturition [17].

The bladder is also an unusual organ because it is functionally "turned off" most of the time, and then turned on in an "all-or-none" manner to eliminate urine. Thus, it behaves differently than other visceral organs such as the heart, blood vessels, and gastrointestinal tract, which receive a tonic autonomic regulation. The ability to "turn on" micturition is facilitated by positive feedback loops in the micturition reflex pathway. In this manner, amplification of bladder afferent activity can activate sufficient efferent excitatory input to the bladder, which in turn initiates a bladder contraction. This positive feedback, mediated in part by supraspinal parasympathetic pathways to the pontine micturition center, is an effective mechanism for promoting efficient bladder emptying and minimizing residual urine.

This positive feedback mechanism, however, also can pose a potentially significant liability. In the presence of neuropathology, this system design can contribute to the emergence of bladder hyperactivity and random urge incontinence. Because of the positive feedback design, loss of central inhibitory controls or sensitization of bladder afferent signaling can lead to the unmasking of involuntary voiding. To balance this design,

nature has provided other mechanisms for inhibitory modulation of the micturition reflex. These more primitive mechanisms reside in the spinal cord, and can be awakened by various somatic and visceral afferent nerve stimulations [22–24]. The spinal organization of these inhibitory mechanisms has been elucidated by electrophysiologic studies in animals [25,26]. The authors hypothesize that these modulatory mechanisms can be activated by SNS in the treatment of overactive bladders.

Afferent and efferent pathways

Efferent outflow to the lower urinary tract can be activated by spinal afferent pathways as well as input from the brain. Afferent input from the pelvic visceral organs and somatic afferent pathways from the perineal muscle and skin are important. Somatic afferent pathways in the pudendal nerves that transmit noxious and nonnoxious information from the genital organs, urethra, prostate, vagina, anal canal, and skin can modulate voiding function [15–17].

Bladder afferent nerves are critical for sending signals of bladder fullness and discomfort to the brain to initiate the micturition reflex. The bladder afferent pathways are composed of two types of axons: small myelinated A-delta fibers and unmyelinated C-fibers. A-delta fibers transmit signals mainly from mechanoreceptors that detect bladder fullness or wall tension. The C-fibers, on the other hand, mainly detect noxious signals and initiate painful sensations. The bladder C-fiber

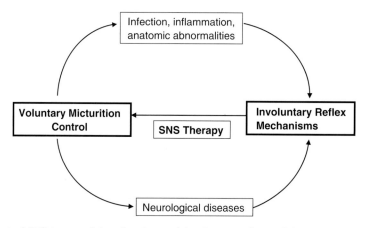

Fig. 1. The concept of SNS is to modulate the abnormal involuntary reflexes of the lower urinary tract and restore voluntary control.

nociceptors perform a similar function and signal the central nervous system when we have an infection or irritative condition in the bladder. C-fiber bladder afferents also have reflex functions to facilitate or trigger voiding [18–20]. This can be viewed as a defense mechanism to eliminate irritants or bacteria. The C-fiber bladder afferents have been implicated in the triggering of reflex bladder hyperactivity associated with neurologic disorders such as spinal cord injury and multiple sclerosis. Capsaicin and its ultrapotent analog, resiniferatoxin, are specific C-fiber afferent neurotoxins undergoing clinical trials for the treatment of lower urinary tract dysfunction relating to C-fiber alterations [15].

Bladder hyperactivity and urinary incontinence are believed to be mediated by the loss of voluntary control of voiding and the appearance of primitive voiding reflex circuitry. This lower urinary tract storage disorder can result from the re-emergence of neonatal reflex patterns that were suppressed during postnatal development or from the formation of new reflex circuits mediated by C-fiber afferents [21]. Under normal conditions, the latter are believed to be mechano-insensitive and unresponsive to bladder distension (hence the term *silent C-fibers*). As a consequence of neurologic or inflammatory diseases or possibly the aging process, however, the silent C-fibers may become sensitized to bladder distension and thus trigger micturition reflexes [18–20]. This type of bladder hyperactivity theoretically could be suppressed by blocking C-fiber afferent activity or by interrupting reflex pathways in the spinal cord by SNS.

Guarding reflexes

An important bladder-to-urethral reflex is mediated by sympathetic efferent pathways to the urethra. This excitatory reflex promotes urethral smooth muscle contraction during the bladder storage phase, and is called the *guarding reflex* [27,28]. This positive reflex is not activated during micturition, but instead when bladder pressure is increased momentarily during events such as a cough or exercise. A second guarding reflex is triggered and amplified by bladder afferent signaling, which synapses with sacral interneurons that in turn activate urethral external sphincter efferent neurons through the pudendal nerve [8]. The activation of pudendal urethral efferents pathways contracts the external urinary sphincter and prevents stress urinary incontinence (Fig. 2).

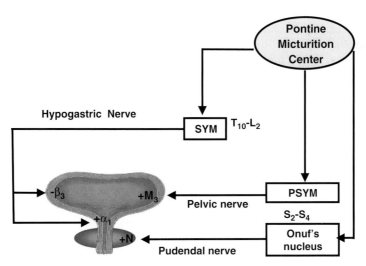

Fig. 2. The key nerves and neurotransmitters of the sympathetic (SYM), parasympathetic (PSYM), and somatic nervous systems involved in bladder control. The parasympathetic nucleus in the sacral cord (S_2–S_4) facilitates bladder emptying by contracting the bladder through the pelvic nerve acting on a muscarinic receptor ($+M_3$) in the detrusor smooth muscle. Hypogastric and pudendal nerves are switched off during micturition. During bladder storage, activation of the somatic pudendal nerve arises from the Onuf's nucleus in S_2–S_4 level that contracts the rhabdosphincter activated by nicotinic receptor ($+N$). In addition, hypogastric nerve activation in the thoracic 10-lumbar-2 (T_{10}-L_2) spinal cord level contracts the internal smooth muscle sphincter by α-1 adrenergic receptor activity, and relaxes the bladder through β-3 adrenergic receptors.

The brain inhibits the guarding reflexes during micturition.

Reflexes that promote micturition

The bladder afferent (A-delta or C-fiber) nerves connect with interneurons in the sacral spinal cord. Interneurons synapse with bladder preganglionic (efferent) parasympathetic neurons to form the bladder-bladder reflex [27–30]. Interneurons activated by bladder afferents also synapse with urethral parasympathetic efferents neurons to form a bladder-urethral reflex. The bladder-bladder reflex is an excitatory reflex that becomes activated with the sensing of the full bladder. Once this reflex is turned "on" it remains on to empty the bladder completely. The bladder-urethral parasympathetic reflex is an inhibitory reflex that induces the smooth muscle of the proximal urethra to relax and the urethral outlet to open reflexively immediately before the onset of a bladder contraction (Fig. 3).

Sacral afferent input can modify micturition reflexes

The guarding and voiding reflexes are activated at different times under different clinical scenarios. Anatomically, however, the sets of neuronal wiring are located closely to each other in the S2–S4 levels of the human spinal cord. Furthermore, both sets of spinal reflex pathways are modulated by several centers in the brain. In this respect, these reflexes can be altered by various neurologic diseases, some of which can unmask

involuntary bladder activity mediated by C-fibers (Fig. 4). SNS modulates these reflexes by altering the afferent signaling and, it is hoped, leading to restoration of voluntary micturition.

Experimental data from animals indicate that somatic afferent input to the sacral spinal cord can modulate the guarding and bladder-bladder reflexes. de Groat [29] has shown that sacral preganglionic outflow to the urinary bladder receives inhibitory inputs from various somatic and visceral afferents, as well as a recurrent inhibitory pathway [22–24]. The experiments also have provided information about the organization of these inhibitory mechanisms [25,26]. Electrical stimulation of somatic afferent in the pudendal nerve elicits inhibitory mechanisms [21]. This is supported by the finding that interneurons in the sacral autonomic nucleus exhibit firing correlated with bladder activity and demonstrate inhibition by activation of somatic afferent pathways. This electrical stimulation of somatic afferent nerves in the sacral spinal roots could inhibit reflex bladder hyperactivity mediated by spinal or supraspinal pathways. In neonatal kittens and rats, micturition as well as defecation are elicited when the mother cat licks the perineal region [21]. In those species, this reflex seems to be the primary stimulus for micturition in the newborn. If the young kitten or rat is separated from its mother, urinary retention occurs.

To induce micturition in humans, the perineal afferents must activate the parasympathetic excitatory input to the bladder but also suppress the urethral sympathetic and sphincter somatic guarding reflexes. Successful suppression of the

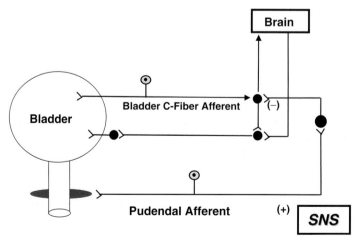

Fig. 3. Pudendal afferent nerve stimulation can inhibit the micturition reflex.

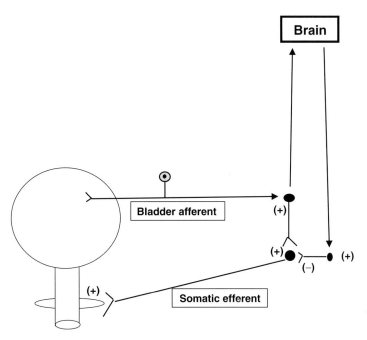

Fig. 4. The guarding reflex prevents urinary incontinence. When there is a sudden increase in intravesical pressure, such as during a cough, the spinal guarding reflex contracts the urinary sphincter to prevent urinary incontinence. The brain turns off the spinal guarding reflex to urinate.

guarding reflexes by SNS enables the enhancement of voiding in the subset of patients who have so-called "idiopathic urinary retention."

The perineal-to-bladder reflex is prominent during the first 4 postnatal weeks. As the kitten approaches the weaning age of 7 to 8 weeks, this perineal-to-bladder reflex dissipates and eventually disappears. In adult animals and humans, perineal stimulation or mechanical stimulation of the sex organs (vagina or penis) have the opposite effect of inhibiting the micturition reflex [17,23,27,28].

Besides the strong evidence from animal research that identified somatic afferent modulation of bladder and urethral reflexes, there are also data from clinical physiologic studies. Such research reinforces the view that stimulation of sacral afferent circuits can modify bladder and urethral sphincter reflexes. For example, functional electrical stimulation offers a favorable nonsurgical treatment for many patients who have detrusor instability. Stimulation techniques typically use surface electrodes, anal and vaginal plug electrodes [2–4], and dorsal penile nerve electrodes [5,6].

The success of pelvic floor electrical stimulation relies on convergence of common visceral and somatic sensory innervation pathways in the central nervous system [31]. By stimulating somatic afferents pathways, it is possible to block the processing of visceral afferent signals being delivered to the same region of the spinal cord. One example is the technique of posterior tibial nerve stimulation. With electrical stimulation of this nerve or its dermatome, it is possible to block sensory afferent inputs from the bladder [32,33]. Olhsson and colleagues [4] report success using electrical somatic nerve stimulation with transvaginal probes in women and transrectal probes in men. Despite a documented average 45% increase in bladder capacity, however, only half of their patients reported a 30% decrease in the frequency of micturition. Fall [2] also reported favorable long-term results of vaginal electrical stimulation in the treatment of refractory detrusor instability and stress urinary incontinence. Seventy-three percent of women who had detrusor instability became asymptomatic during treatment, whereas 45% remained free of symptoms after discontinuation of therapy. Many patients, however, required up to 6 months of therapy before benefit was apparent.

How sacral nerve stimulation works

The authors hypothesize that the effects of SNS depend on electrical stimulation of somatic afferent axons in the spinal roots, which in turn modulate voiding and continence reflex pathways in the central nervous system. The afferent system is the most likely target because beneficial effects can be elicited at intensities of stimulation that do not activate movements of striated muscles [34–36].

Urinary retention and dysfunctional voiding can be resolved by inhibition of the guarding reflexes. Detrusor hyperreflexia can be suppressed by two mechanisms: (1) direct inhibition of bladder preganglionic neurons and (2) inhibition of interneuronal transmission in the afferent limb of the micturition reflex.

How do sacral somatic afferents alter lower urinary tract reflexes to promote voiding? In adults, brain pathways are necessary to turn off sphincter and urethral guarding reflexes to allow efficient bladder emptying. Thus spinal cord injury produces bladder sphincter dyssynergia and inefficient bladder emptying by eliminating the brain mechanisms (Fig. 5). This also may occur after more subtle neurologic lesions in patients who have idiopathic urinary retention, such as after a bout of prostatitis or urinary tract infection.

As discussed previously, tactile stimulation of the perineum in the newborn cat also inhibits the bladder-sympathetic reflex component of the guarding reflex mechanism. Before the development of brain control, the pudendal nerve can initiate efficient voiding by activating bladder

efferent pathways and turning off the excitatory pathways to the urethral outlet [15,16,18]. The authors hypothesize that SNS can elicit similar responses in patients who have urinary retention, turning off excitatory outflow to the urethral outlet and promoting bladder emptying. Because sphincter activity can generate afferent input to the spinal cord that can inhibit reflex bladder activity, an indirect benefit of suppressing sphincter reflexes would be a facilitation of bladder emptying function. This also may be useful in this patient population.

Conversely, how do sacral afferents also play a role in the inhibition of the overactive bladder? Several reflex mechanisms may be involved in the SNS suppression of bladder hyperactivity. Afferent pathways projecting to the sacral cord can inhibit bladder reflexes in animals and humans through two means: (1) by inhibiting the sacral interneuronal transmission and (2) by direct inhibition of bladder preganglionic neurons of the efferent limb of the micturition reflex circuit. The source of afferent input may be somatic, visceral, or both: namely, sphincter muscles, distal colon, rectum, anal canal, vagina, uterine cervix, and cutaneous innervation from the perineum.

Of the two mechanisms responsible for somatic and visceral afferent inhibition of bladder reflexes, the suppression of interneuronal transmission in

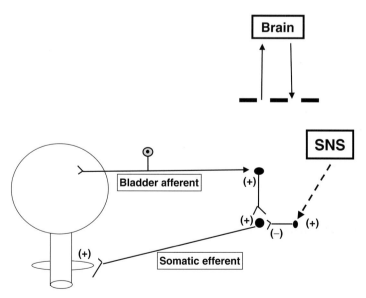

Fig. 5. In cases of neurologic diseases, the brain cannot turn off the spinal guarding reflex to urinate and retention can occur. SNS can restore voluntary micturition in cases of voiding dysfunction and urinary retention by inhibiting the spinal guarding reflex.

the bladder reflex pathway is believed to be involved most commonly in SNS [18,37,38]. It is believed that this inhibition occurs in part on the ascending limb of the micturition reflex and therefore blocks the transfer of signaling input from the bladder to the pontine micturition center. This action would prevent involuntary (reflex) micturition, but not suppress voluntary voiding necessarily. This is the clinical scenario typically observed in SNS therapy of overactive bladder.

The preservation of volitional voiding function suggests that the descending excitatory efferent pathways from the brain to the sacral parasympathetic preganglionic neurons are not inhibited. This latter mechanism would be more effective in turning off micturition reflexes because it would suppress directly firing in the motor outflow from the spinal cord. This can be induced by electrical stimulation of the pudendal nerve or by mechanical stimulation of the anal canal and distal bowel. As discussed, however, it also would be expected to block voluntary and involuntary voiding nonselectively. Therefore, this inhibitory pathway seems to play a lesser role in SNS' mechanism of action. Experience has shown that SNS performed

for either voiding dysfunction or overactive bladder syndrome typically allows patients to retain normal voiding mechanisms (Box 1).

Summary

The authors believe that the principles underlying the multiple possible SNS mechanisms of action can be summarized as somatic afferent inhibition of sensory processing in the spinal cord. Regardless of whether the lower urinary tract dysfunction involves storage versus emptying abnormalities, the pudendal afferent signaling serves as a common crossroads in the neurologic wiring of the system. Not only can pudendal afferent input turn on voiding reflexes by suppressing the guarding reflex pathways, pudendal afferent input to the sacral spinal cord also can turn off supraspinally mediated hyperactive voiding by blocking ascending sensory pathway inputs.

For these reasons, SNS can take advantage of the complex neurologic pathways described and offer successful treatment for a seemingly disparate group of lower urinary tract pathologies. SNS is a urologic technique that has proved safe and minimally invasive, and it holds great promise for many patients who have lower urinary tract dysfunction.

Box 1. Possible mechanisms of sacral nerve stimulation

- Inhibits postganglionic neurons directly
- May inhibit primary afferents presynaptically
- Inhibits spinal tract neurons involved in the micturition reflex
- Inhibits interneurons involved in spinal segmental reflexes
- May suppress indirectly guarding reflexes by turning off bladder afferent input to internal sphincter sympathetic or external urethral sphincter interneurons
- Postganglionic stimulation can activate postganglionic neurons directly and induce bladder activity (induce voiding), but at the same time can turn off bladder-to-bladder reflex by inhibiting afferent-interneuronal transmission

---

References

[1] Schmidt RA. Treatment of unstable bladder. Urology 1991;37:28.
[2] Fall M. Electrical pelvic floor stimulation for the control of detrusor instability. Neurourol Urodyn 1985;4:329.
[3] Janez J, Plevnik S, Suhet P. Urethral and bladder responses to anal electrical stimulation. J Urol 1979;122:192.
[4] Ohlsson BL, Fall M, Frankenbers-Sommar S. Effects of external and direct pudendal nerve maximal electrical stimulation in the treatment of the uninhibited overactive bladder. Br J Urol 1989;64:374.
[5] Walter JS, Wheeler JS, Robinson CJ, et al. Inhibiting the hyperreflexic bladder with electrical stimulation in a spinal animal model. Neurourol Urodyn 1993;12:241.
[6] Wheeler JS, Walter JS. Bladder inhibition by dorsal penile nerve stimulation in spinal cord injured patients. J Urol 1992;147:100.
[7] Bosch JLHR, Groen J. Sacral (S3) segmental nerve stimulation as a treatment for urge incontinence in patients with detrusor instability: results of chronic

electrical stimulation using an implantable prosthesis. J Urol 1995;154:504.

[8] Shaker HS, Hassouna M. Sacral nerve root neuromodulation: an effective treatment for refractory urge incontinence. J Urol 1998;159:1516.

[9] Shaker HS, Hassouna M. Sacral root neuromodulation in idiopathic nonobstructive chronic urinary retention. J Urol 1998;159:1476.

[10] Vapnek JM, Schmidt RA. Restoration of voiding in chronic urinary retention using neuroprosthesis. World J Urol 1991;9:142.

[11] Juenemann KP, Lue TF, Schmidt RA, et al. Clinical significance of sacral and pudendal nerve anatomy. J Urol 1988;139:74

[12] Schmidt RA, Tanagho EA. Feasibility of controlled micturition through electric stimulation. Urol Int 1979;34:199.

[13] Schmidt RA, Sennm E, Tanagho EA. Functional evaluation of sacral nerve root integrity. Report of a technique. Urology 1990;35:388.

[14] Tanagho EA, Schmidt RA. Electrical stimulation in the clinical management of the neurogenic bladder. J Urol 1988;140:1331.

[15] Yoshimura N, de Groat WC. Neural control of the lower urinary tract. Int J Urol 1997;4:111.

[16] de Groat WC. Central nervous system control of micturition. In: O'Donnell PD, editor. Urinary incontinence. St. Louis (MO): Mosby; 1997. p. 33–47.

[17] de Groat WC, Araki I, Vizzard MA, et al. Developmental and injury induced plasticity in the micturition reflex pathway. Behav Brain Res 1997;92:127.

[18] Kruse MN, de Groat WC. Spinal pathways mediate coordinated bladder/urethral sphincter activity during reflex micturition in normal and spinal cord injured neonatal rats Neurosci Lett 1993;152:141.

[19] Cheng CI, Ma CP, de Groat WC. Effect of capsaicin on micturition and associated reflexes in rats. Am J Physiol 1993;34:R132.

[20] Cheng CI, Ma CP, de Groat WC. Effect of capsaicin on micturition and associated reflexes in chronic spinal rats Brain Res 1995;378:40.

[21] de Groat WC. Changes in the organization of the micturition reflex pathway of the cat after transection of the spinal cord. In: Veraa RP, Grafstein B, editors. Cellular mechanisms for recovery from nervous systems injury: a conference report. Exp Neurol 1981;71:22.

[22] de Groat WC, Ryall RW. The identification and antidromic responses of sacral preganglionic parasympathetic neurons. J Physiol (Lond) 1968;196:533.

[23] de Groat WC, Ryall RW. Recurrent inhibition in sacral parasympathetic pathways to the bladder. J Physiol (Lond) 1968;196:579

[24] de Groat WC. Nervous control of the urinary bladder of the cat. Brain Res 1975;87:201.

[25] de Groat WC. Excitation and inhibition of sacral parasympathetic neurons by visceral and cutaneous stimuli in the cat. Brain Res 1971;33:499.

[26] de Groat WC. Mechanisms underlying recurrent inhibition in the sacral parasympathetic outflow to the urinary bladder. J Physiol 1976;257:503.

[27] de Groat WC, Vizzard MA, Araki I, et al. Spinal interneurons and preganglionic neurons in sacral autonomic reflex pathways. In: Holstege G, Bandler R, Saper C, editors. The emotional motor system. Prog Brain Res 1996;107:97.

[28] de Groat WC, Nadelhaft I, Milne RJ, et al. Organization of the sacral parasympathetic reflex pathways to the urinary bladder and large intestine. J Auton Nerv Syst 1981;3:135.

[29] de Groat WC. Inhibitory mechanisms in the sacral reflex pathways to the urinary bladder. In: Ryall RW, Kelly JS, editors. Iontophoresis and transmitter mechanisms in the mammalian central nervous system. Amsterdam: Elsevier; 1978. p. 366–8.

[30] de Groat WC. Mechanisms underlying the recovery of lower urinary tract function following spinal cord injury. Paraplegia 1995;33:493.

[31] Morrison JFB. Neural connections between the lower urinary tract and the spinal cord. In: Torrens M, Morrison JFB, editors. The physiology of the lower urinary tract. London: Springer Verlag; 1987. p. 53–85.

[32] McGuire EJ, Shi-Chun Z, Horwinski R, et al. Treatment of motor and sensory detrusor instability by electrical stimulation. J Urol 1983;129:78.

[33] Crocker M, Doleys DM, Dolce JJ. Transcutaneous electrical nerve stimulation in urinary retention. South Med J 1985;78:1515.

[34] Thon WF, Baskin LS, Jonas U, et al. Surgical principles of sacral foramen electrode implantation. World J Urol 1991;9:133.

[35] Vadusek DB, Light JK, Liddy JM. Detrusor inhibition induced by stimulation of pudendal nerve afferents. Neurourol Urodyn 1986;5:381.

[36] de Groat WC, Kruse MN, Vizzard MA, et al. Modification of urinary bladder function after neural injury. In: Seil F, editor. Neuronal regeneration, reorganization, and repair New York: Lippincott-Raven Publishers; 1997. p. 347–64. Advances in Neurology, vol 72.

[37] Kruse MN, Noto H, Roppolo JR, et al. Pontine control of the urinary bladder and external urethral sphincter in the rat. Brain Res 1990;532:182.

[38] de Groat WC, Theobald RJ. Reflex activation of sympathetic pathways to vesical smooth muscle and parasympathetic ganglia by electrical stimulation of vesical afferents. J Physiol 1976;259:223.

ELSEVIER
SAUNDERS

Urol Clin N Am 32 (2005) 19–26

UROLOGIC
CLINICS
of North America

Selecting Patients for Sacral Nerve Stimulation

Steven W. Siegel, MD

*Center for Continence Care, Metropolitan Urologic Specialists, 360 Sherman Ave, Suite 450,
St. Paul, MN 55102, USA*

Although sacral nerve stimulation (SNS) has become an accepted treatment modality for chronic voiding dysfunction, there still are no clear predictive factors, and patient selection remains largely empiric. Which patients are appropriate candidates for SNS? The answer becomes easier as a greater familiarity and comfort level with the therapy is achieved. Patients who have symptoms of voiding dysfunction that are not helped by other measures should be considered.

There are two keys to patient selection: first, to define the patient problem in terms of the voiding behaviors and pelvic floor muscle function instead of diagnostic labels that are often organ-based; and second, to think of the trial phase of SNS as a completely reversible diagnostic procedure with little risk to the patient. A therapy trial (percutaneous nerve evaluation or staged implant) is the ultimate predictive test for patient selection. Once this approach is adopted, the response of the patient to a trial of therapy becomes the ultimate answer, often with dramatic emphasis.

Profile of an ideal patient for sacral nerve stimulation

History

The patient is a middle-aged woman who complained of urinary frequency of up to 20 voids in 24 hours. The stream was often inefficient, with small voided volumes, and a sensation of incomplete emptying. The degree of urgency was out of proportion to the voided volume, but she could hold it if she had to. She had rare episodes of incontinence. The symptoms were present for several years, and were not helped by various anticholinergic agents. She felt as though her life revolved around the bathroom. There were associated complaints of suprapubic pain or pressure with bladder fullness, and if she tried to hold it, the pain increased. She had a previous total abdominal hysterectomy with bilateral salpingo-oophorectomy for endometriosis, and afterward developed some pain attributed to adhesions in the right lower quadrant. She believed her bladder symptoms became prominent after the hysterectomy. There was also a significant problem of irritable bowel, with marked constipation. She complained of pain with intercourse, and in certain activities, such as riding a bike or sitting.

On physical examination, she was noted to have dull suprapubic tenderness, and obvious tenderness upon palpation of the levators, with transvaginal palpation on the right side reproducing her right lower quadrant pain. On digital rectal examination there was hard stool present in the rectal ampulla. The resting tone of the levator muscles was tense, and there was no ability to relax them. She had poor ability to identify and contract the pelvic floor muscles, and performed a facial grimace, abdominal strain, and pelvic tilt while trying.

Evaluation

The postvoid residual was 75 mL, and there was discomfort upon catheterization. Her urinalysis and cystoscopy were unremarkable. A pelvic ultrasound was negative for a focal abnormality. A urodynamic examination showed a volitional volume of 145 mL, with a hypersensitive filling pattern. There was normal compliance and no evidence of uninhibited detrusor activity. There

E-mail address: pnedoc@comcast.net

was spastic pelvic floor muscle electromyogram (EMG) activity measured by patch perianal electrodes throughout the filling phase, and during voiding, she relaxed incompletely, and attempted to void by abdominal straining. The flow pattern was intermittent and prolonged on the free-flow study and on instrumented flow. A moderate residual was present.

Treatment

A trial of a tricyclic antidepressant, combined with a fiber supplement, decreased her pain and constipation, but her frequency persisted. Her problem was defined as "urinary frequency and urgency with pelvic pain due to pelvic floor muscle spasticity." A course of pelvic floor muscle EMG biofeedback was not completed because of poor compliance, and the inability of the patient to learn to relax her pelvic floor.

Staged sacral nerve stimulation trial

A staged trial of SNS was performed, with placement of a tined lead under local anesthesia with sedation. The lead was placed at the S3 level on the right because her pain was lateralizing. During the lead placement, the patient felt the stimulation as a comfortable vibration and pulling in the vaginal area. She felt a "release" of the pressure in the suprapubic area. Over the ensuing 30-day trial period, the patient's diaries reflected a dramatic decrease in the voiding frequency, along with a corresponding increase in the voided volumes. There was also a subjective improvement in the stream force and sense of complete bladder evacuation. She noted complete resolution of her suprapubic pressure and right lower quadrant pain. She began having daily bowel movements within days of initiating the trial, a complete change from her prior pattern of bowel function. The patient considered the therapeutic trial to be a dramatic improvement, and received an implantable pulse generator as a second-stage completion procedure. She has continued to experience improvement of her symptoms over several years.

Indications for sacral nerve stimulation therapy

The US Food and Drug Administration (FDA) approved SNS for intractable urge incontinence in 1997, and for urgency-frequency and nonobstructive urinary retention in 1999. Later, the labeling was changed to include "overactive bladder" as an appropriate diagnostic category. Patients in these groups are appropriate for SNS when they have chronic symptoms that significantly affect quality of life, and conservative treatments have been unsuccessful [1,2].

Overactive bladder

Overactive bladder represents a mixed group of disorders with a common set of voiding behaviors, including urinary urgency-frequency and urge incontinence. In most instances, the etiology is deemed idiopathic. A behavioral component or pelvic floor muscle dysfunction is commonly present. There frequently is evidence of pelvic floor muscle spasticity on examination and on urodynamic study. The urodynamic study may or may not demonstrate uninhibited detrusor contractions. There may have been a triggering event such as a pelvic surgery (eg, surgery for stress incontinence) or trauma. As a rule, patients who are appropriate candidates for SNS are neurologically normal, and have no structural abnormality of the bladder (eg, scarring from radiation therapy, or a diverticulum).

Neurogenic disorders

Patients who have defined neurologic abnormalities such as multiple sclerosis (MS) or partial cord injury also may benefit, but studies in this population of patients have been few. When faced with the alternative of an indwelling catheter or urinary diversion, it may be reasonable to consider a diagnostic trial of SNS. Patients who have disorders such as peripheral neuropathy, a cord lesion, MS, parkinsonism, or myelodysplasia are not ideal candidates. Patients who have MS, for example, were excluded from original trials leading to FDA approval because of the potential for the underlying condition to change [3]. If this were to occur, the FDA may have questioned the effectiveness of the therapy. SNS helps patients who have MS [4], however, and in some cases, may be the most appropriate option.

Interstitial cystitis and pelvic pain

Interstitial cystitis (IC) per se is not an FDA-approved indication for SNS, but as in the patient example, one could define a set of symptoms characteristic of IC as "urinary frequency and urgency with pelvic pain." By using a diagnostic label based on objective voiding behaviors, patients who have IC readily fit into the approved diagnostic criteria. Although isolated symptoms of pelvic floor muscle dysfunction, pelvic pain, or bowel dysfunction are not indications for the therapy, they are commonly present in patients who are otherwise candidates for SNS, and frequently improve along with the urinary complaints if the therapy is otherwise successful [5–10].

Nonobstructive urinary retention

Nonobstructive urinary retention also is often understood as idiopathic. It may arise following an otherwise uneventful pelvic surgery such as a hysterectomy or sling procedure, or result from conscious or unconscious holding. By definition, patients who are candidates for SNS have no urodynamic evidence of obstruction [11]. Physicians who would not hesitate to do a transurethral resection of the prostate or a sling lysis on such a patient may not have considered or are undecided about the potential value of a diagnostic SNS trial.

Pelvic floor muscle dysfunction

As in the case example, pelvic floor muscle dysfunction is a key component of common urologic complaints. It is a unifying feature of symptoms such as urgency-frequency, urge incontinence, and idiopathic urinary retention, and the finding often is associated with bowel dysfunction and pelvic pain. The pelvic floor muscle behavior can be assessed readily during routine physical examination, as well as urodynamic assessment. Conservative therapies should be aimed at improving the range of pelvic floor motion from a comfortable, relaxed baseline to a coordinated, sustainable, and strong maximal contraction.

How common is pelvic floor muscle dysfunction? In a study by Bourcier [12], 78% of 316 postpartum females had moderate to poor function of the pelvic floor muscles. Bo and colleagues [13] noted that one third of all patients could not contract the pelvic floor upon verbal command. In another study, Bourcier and Juras [14] noted that 22% of postpartum females performed a Valsalva maneuver when asked to contract the pelvic floor muscles. Patients who cannot identify the pelvic floor muscles, and who do not have a range of motion from coordinated relaxation to efficient contraction, are unable to find the voluntary "on-off" switch to the bladder, and are prone to voiding dysfunction. These patients are

candidates for SNS when conservative methods of management are unsuccessful [15].

Failed prior conservative therapy

Patients who are candidates for an SNS trial should have undergone a trial of conservative therapy first. Conservative therapies include medications such as anticholinergics, tricyclics, and striated and smooth muscle relaxants. It is up to the individual physician whether treatments specific for IC are appropriate, and for how long. Behavioral techniques include behavior modification, pelvic floor exercises, and EMG biofeedback (Fig. 1). There also may be a role for physical therapy for sacro iliac joint dysfunction, pubic shear, or myofascial release. Candidates for SNS also may have failed a trial of external stimulation, such as transvaginal or transanal pelvic floor stimulation, percutaneous tibial nerve stimulation, or extracorporeal magnetic innervation. In the case of urge incontinence, they would otherwise be candidates for intravesical botox injection, augmentation cystoplasy, denervation techniques, or urinary diversion.

Contraindications

In patients who have anatomic changes such as bony abnormalities of the sacrum, transforaminal access may be difficult or impossible (Fig. 2). Patients for whom future MRI studies will be critical also potentially are contraindicated. Patients with mental incapacity rendering them incapable of operating the device or giving appropriate feedback regarding the comfort of stimulation are also poor candidates. Patients who use other stimulation devices, such as a cardiac pacemaker, also are potentially contraindicated, unless, with simultaneous monitoring, it can be demonstrated that there is no interference with the cardiac device during acute stimulation. Finally, patients who have undergone an unsuccessful trial of SNS (failed test stimulation) are inappropriate for permanent treatment with this method.

Clinical evaluation of voiding dysfunction

The tools necessary for proper evaluation of patients who have voiding dysfunction are readily available. They involve a careful history, physical examination, routine tests such as urinalysis and urine culture, simple diagnostic tests such as pelvic ultrasound and cystoscopy, and the use of diaries

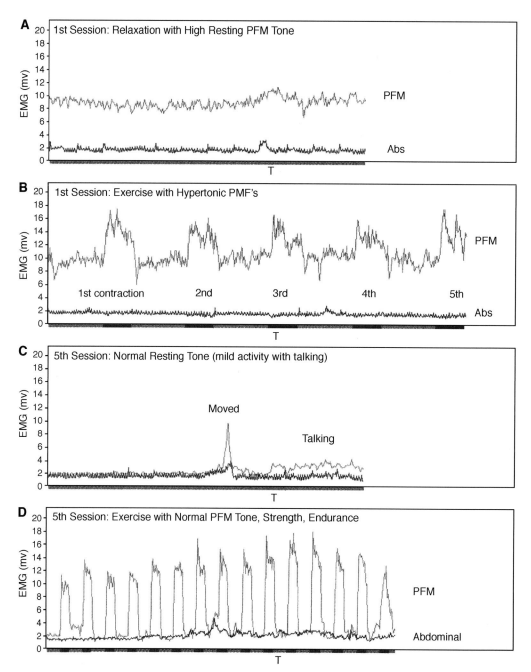

Fig. 1. (*A*) Graph from the first session of a course of pelvic floor muscle (PFM) EMG biofeedback. The patient complained of urinary urgency and frequency that was not controlled by anticholinergic medications. During relaxation, the patient demonstrates increased PFM tone. Abdominal muscle EMG activity is measured as a control. A patient should be able to relax the pelvic floor muscle to a baseline <2 μV. (*B*) During exercise, the patient can isolate the PFMs well, but has a decreased range of motion from maximal relaxation to maximal contraction. (*C*) The same patient 6 weeks later during her fifth session. Here, the PFM resting tone has normalized during relaxation. (*D*) In the same timeframe, during exercise, the patient has maintained a normal baseline PFM tone, and has improved her strength and endurance during contraction. The patient's symptoms were ultimately well controlled with conservative therapy.

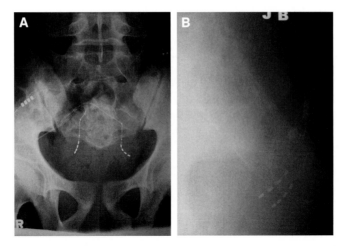

Fig. 2. Anterior-posterior (*A*) and lateral (*B*) sacral radiographs showing evidence of a sacral deformity. The patient had a presacral teratoma resected in infancy and a lifetime of voiding dysfunction, including retention requiring intermittent self-catheterization. Sensation and neurologic examination were normal; there was no sexual dysfunction or gait abnormality. The bony deformity is a relative contraindication to SNS because the normal landmarks are not present. He experienced spontaneous voiding with no residuals during the staged trial.

to objectify appropriate voiding variables. A urodynamic examination to identify abnormal pelvic floor muscle function is also of great help (Fig. 3).

History

The history focuses on the primary voiding variables such as the frequency and severity of urge-incontinent episodes and the number of pads used per 24-hour period. For urgency-frequency syndrome, the number of voids, the voided volumes, and the degree of urgency are assessed, and in patients who experience inefficient voiding or urinary retention, the amount voided versus catheterized volumes per 24 hours and the patient's sense of completeness of evacuation are fathomed. Associated symptoms such as pelvic pain and bowel and sexual symptoms also are assessed. As in the case example, they are often a part of the clinical presentation of patients who have voiding dysfunction who are candidates for SNS, and these symptoms may improve with successful treatment. As an extension of the history, a voiding diary is invaluable to objectify the patient's complaints.

Physical examination

The physical examination is an extremely important part of the assessment of patients who

have voiding dysfunction. Evidence of high-tone pelvic floor muscle dysfunction is often present in patients who do well with SNS. It begins by looking at the patient (Fig. 4). Often the patient is standing because it hurts to sit, or, if they are sitting, they frequently balance in such a way as to keep direct pressure off their pelvic floor muscles. These signals of important underlying pathology are apparent immediately.

The physical examination also involves the routine determination of the presence of hypermobility, stress incontinence, and pelvic prolapse. In addition, a neurourologic examination should be performed to check for saddle sensation, sphincter tone, and bulbocavernosus reflex. A residual urine volume needs to be determined. Tenderness upon catheterization is an important finding that should be noted.

The rectal examination is a key aspect of the physical examination of any patient who has voiding dysfunction. Levator function and tone must be assessed. It may be normal, absent, or weak (a rare finding among patients who have voiding dysfunction) or spastic and tender (which is more common). Often these patients display an increased resting tone, and a functionally frozen pelvic floor, as in the case example. The author often notes that after placing an examining finger in the rectum and asking the patient to squeeze the finger, the patient reaches around with his or her hand to grab the finger. This indicates a lack of

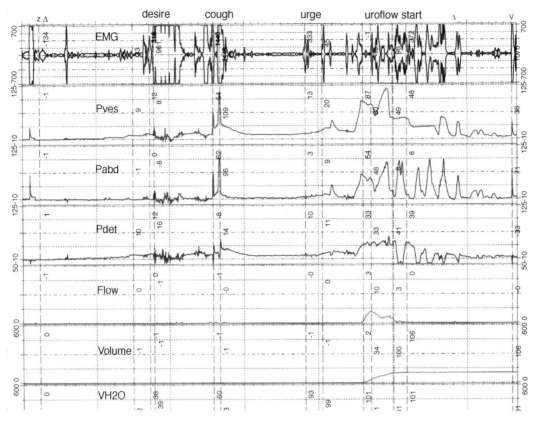

Fig. 3. Urodynamic study of a patient who had urinary frequency, urgency, and pelvic pain showing a diminished volitional capacity (100 mL) with uninhibited detrusor contractions. It is important to look at both filling and voiding phases of bladder function. There is a detrusor contraction with voiding, and the patient exhibits dysfunctional voiding behavior with incomplete relaxation of the pelvic floor muscles and abdominal straining. The flow pattern of such patients often is intermittent or "saw-toothed."

conscious connection between the patient and the pelvic floor muscles.

Pelvic floor muscle electromyogram

Another method of demonstrating inappropriate pelvic floor muscle behavior is by measuring pelvic floor muscle EMG activity. This typically is not done during physical examination but, instead, during pelvic floor muscle rehabilitation using EMG biofeedback (see Fig. 1). As in the case example, a patient who demonstrates abnormal pelvic floor muscle behavior, and cannot improve sufficiently with biofeedback or pelvic floor muscle physical therapy, is a good candidate for an SNS trial.

Urodynamic assessment

Urodynamic examination also can be tailored to demonstrate abnormal pelvic floor muscle

behavior (see Fig. 3). Typically there are several components, including a simple or uninstrumented uroflow followed by residual check. This serves as a snapshot of "normal" voiding before the more invasive portion of the study begins, and should be compared with the patient's estimation of normal voiding and to the instrumented flow study to assess its accuracy. A medium fill rate cystometrogram followed by an instrumented pressure flow study are performed next, and the pelvic floor muscle EMG behavior is measured during the filling and voiding phases using patch perianal EMG electrodes. The primary purpose of the urodynamic evaluation is to rule out treatable causes of urinary incontinence or obstruction. Patients who have idiopathic retention typically have normal neurologic examinations and intact sensation. Their urodynamic examinations often demonstrate awareness of filling, and normal capacity and compliance. There may be an

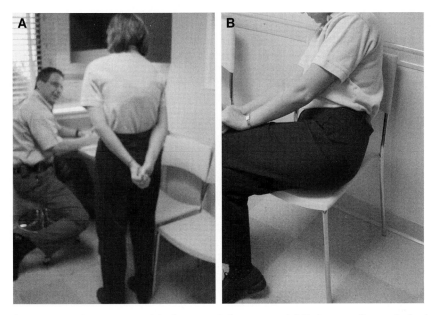

Fig. 4. A patient's posture demonstrates pelvic floor muscle hypertonus. (*A*) Patient standing at the beginning of the encounter. (*B*) Patient sitting "off-center" to keep pressure off her pelvic floor muscles. What would her pelvic floor muscle examination likely show?

increase in EMG signaling from the striated sphincter, with inability to relax the sphincter during voiding attempts. There is often no evidence of a detrusor contraction during voiding attempts, and evidence of bladder outlet obstruction must be ruled out.

Summary

Patient selection for SNS remains empiric. A key is to think of voiding dysfunctions in terms of voiding behaviors and pelvic floor muscle function, not organ-based labels. Patients who have intractable urinary frequency, urgency, urge incontinence, or idiopathic urinary retention should be considered as prime candidates. Evidence of high-tone pelvic floor muscle dysfunction also may be demonstrated on routine physical examination, as well as diagnostic studies such as pelvic-floor EMG. A successful trial stimulation remains the best indicator for patient selection, and should be used as a routine diagnostic test among patients who have chronic, life-altering voiding complaints that cannot be resolved adequately by medications or behavioral interventions.

References

[1] Siegel SW, Catanzaro F, Dijkema H, et al. Long-term results of a multicenter study on sacral nerve stimulation for treatment of urinary urge incontinence, urgency-frequency, and retention. Urology 2000;4(56 Suppl 1):87–91.

[2] Abrams P, Blaivas J, Fowler C, et al. The role of neuromodulation in the management of urinary urge incontinence. BJU Int 2003;91(4):355–9.

[3] Hassouna M, Siegel S, Nyeholt A, et al. Sacral neuromodulation in the treatment of urgency-frequency symptoms: a multicenter study on efficacy and safety. J Urol 2000;163:1849–54.

[4] Bosch J, Groen J. Treatment of refractory urge urinary incontinence with sacral spinal nerve stimulation in multiple sclerosis patients. Lancet 1996; 348(9029):717–9.

[5] Lukban J, Whitmore K, Sant G. Current management of interstitial cystitis. Urol Clin North Am 2002;29:649–60.

[6] Everaert K, Devulder J, De Muynck M, et al. The pain cycle: implications for the diagnosis and treatment of pelvic pain syndromes. Int Urogynecol J Pelvic Floor Dysfunct 2001;12:9–14.

[7] Siegel S, Paszkiewicz E, Kirkpatrick C, et al. Sacral nerve stimulation in patients with chronic intractable pelvic pain. J Urol 2001;166(5):1742–5.

[8] Comiter C. Sacral neuromodulation for the symptomatic treatment of refractory interstial cystitis: a prospective study. J Urol 2003;169:1369–73.

[9] Peters K. Sacral neuromodulation decreases narcotic requirements in refractory interstitial cystitis. BJU Int 2004;93(6):777–9.

[10] Peters K. Sacral neuromodulation for the treatment of refractory interstitial cystitis: outcomes based on

technique. Int Urogynecol J Pelvic Floor Dysfunct 2003;14(4):223–8.

[11] Everaert K, Plancke H, Lefevre F, et al. The urodynamic evaluation of neuromodulation in patients with voiding dysfunction. Br J Urol 1997;79(5): 702–7.

[12] Bourcier A. Physical therapy for female pelvic floor disorders. Curr Opin Obstet Gynecol 1994;4:331–5.

[13] Bo K. Nonpharmacologic treatments for overactive bladder-pelvic floor exercises. Urology 2000; 55(Suppl 5):7–11.

[14] Bourcier A, Juras J. Nonsurgical therapy for stress incontinence. Urol Clin North Am 1995;22:613–27.

[15] Aboseif S, Tamaddon K, Chalfin S, et al. Sacral neuromodulation as an effective treatment for refractory pelvic floor dysfunction. Urology 2002;60(1):52–6.

ELSEVIER
SAUNDERS

Urol Clin N Am 32 (2005) 27–35

UROLOGIC
CLINICS
of North America

Surgical Techniques of Sacral Implantation

Toby C. Chai, MD, FACS

Division of Urology, University of Maryland School of Medicine, 22 South Greene Street,
S8D18, Baltimore, MD 21201, USA

S3 nerve stimulation has been used to treat voiding dysfunction ranging from urge incontinence and frequency-urgency syndrome to idiopathic urinary retention. The effect of S3 neurostimulation is to modulate bladder behavior, whether it is to enhance storage or emptying ability. Neuromodulation refers to the effects of electrical stimulation (neurostimulation) on the nerves resulting in either excitation or inhibition of the effector or target organ, such as the bladder. Neuromodulation and neurostimulation are often used interchangeably, although the definitions are not exactly equivalent.

Schmidt et al [1], who pioneered methods in sacral neurostimulation, observed that patients who were undergoing S3 nerve evaluation had improvement of their voiding symptoms. Medtronic (Minneapolis, MN) developed InterStim therapy based on Schmidt's observations. InterStim was approved by the Food and Drug Administration for use in urge incontinence in 1997 and approval for frequency-urgency syndrome and idiopathic urinary retention indications followed shortly afterward.

The technique of InterStim, when first introduced, was a two-step procedure. The first step was evaluating a patient's bladder symptoms in response to S3 stimulation during a test stimulation period of 3 to 4 days by a temporary wire placed percutaneously into S3 foramen and electrically stimulated by an external stimulator (this step was called the percutaneous nerve evaluation). If the patient had significant improvement in symptoms (<50% reduction of bladder

symptoms, such as voiding frequency, number of incontinent episodes, number of pad used, urgency scale, postvoid residual volume, or number of self-catheterization events), then he or she was a candidate for the second step, which was simultaneous surgical implantation of both a permanent S3 lead and a pulse generator for chronic S3 neurostimulation.

The percutaneous nerve evaluation was typically performed using local anesthesia and without fluoroscopic guidance. S3 foramen was localized using a combination of palpation and assessment of patient's motor and sensory responses to electrical stimulation of the foramen needle. The temporary lead, introduced through a foramen needle, was taped to the patients and often migrated out of the S3 foramen. The second step, or implantation step, occurred in the operating room with the patient under general anesthesia. Unfortunately, there was no reliable way of ensuring that the placement of the implantable S3 lead replicated the exact location of temporary lead. Furthermore, the temporary and implantable leads were of different construction. These factors made the replication of efficacy between the temporary and permanent leads unpredictable. There were several different techniques used for implantation of the permanent S3 leads. These modifications included fixation to the dorsal sacral periosteum [2], anchoring to lumbosacral fascia [3], or a small sacral laminectomy to expose directly the S3 nerve roots [4]. The first two techniques did not require laminectomy and the leads were placed into the S3 foramen with or without angiocatheter guidance. After the lead was implanted, then the implantable pulse generator (IPG) was placed in the anterior abdominal wall.

E-mail address: tchai@smail.umaryland.edu

Surgical modifications

Implantation of implantable pulse generator in buttock region

One of the earliest modifications of InterStim therapy was to change the location of where the pulse generator is implanted. As originally described, the IPG was to be placed in the anterior abdominal wall. This required the patient to be turned over during the operative case. The S3 lead was first implanted with the patient in a prone position. After the lead was implanted, the patient was turned over to a supine position or a modified flank position to access the abdominal wall. The location of the IPG was modified to the upper buttock almost as soon as InterStim was introduced in 1997 and results from a multicenter trial using a buttock approach were published in 2001 [5]. This modification allowed the patient to remain in one position and eliminated an incision in the abdominal wall.

Fluoroscopic guidance for S3 lead placement

The original techniques for S3 localization included palpation of the sciatic notch, observation for least curved portion of the sacrum, and measurement of distance from the coccyx. These techniques became more difficult for obese patients or those without palpable landmarks. The introduction of the "cross-hair" fluoroscopic technique for S3 localization was first published in 2001 [3]. The intent of the fluoroscopy was not meant to "see" the S3 foramen, but rather to help the surgeon identify a specific region to start percutaneous access of S3 foramen. More importantly, the use of lateral imaging helped determine the depth required for implanting the S3 lead [3]. Urologists are familiar in the use of fluoroscopy in stone surgery and the application of fluoroscopy to sacral neuromodulation surgery was quickly accepted. What fluoroscopy did was ultimately allow for the evolution of an open lead implantation to a totally percutaneous approach (see next section).

Percutaneous technique in S3 lead implantation

The S3 lead implant required an open incision with several options for the lead anchoring. One of the major differences between urologists in the United States and Europe was whether a sacral laminectomy was performed. Urologists in the United States did not perform laminectomies and the S3 leads were introduced through S3 foramen manually or with a guide and anchored to the sacral periosteum or lumbosacral fascial [2,3]. European centers have used limited laminectomies to expose the S3 nerve roots [4]. Because of the invasiveness of all of these techniques, several modifications occurred to simplify lead implantation. The lumbosacral anchoring technique was the first modification [3]. This approach required only an open dissection down to the lumbosacral fascia without requiring exposure of the sacral periosteum; the lead was introduced into the S3 foramen using a 14-guage angiocath guide and a slideable anchor was used to fix the lead to the fascia.

The concept of percutaneously implanting a lead into S3 foramen was operationalized with the introduction of the tined S3 lead [6]. The percutaneous implantation technique borrows from the Seldinger technique to insert a permanent lead with tined plastic hooks into the S3 foramen. Use of a special introducer is required for this technique. Lateral fluoroscopy, adapted from previously described modification [3], is used to implant the tined lead properly.

Staged implantation

The original method of InterStim followed two steps: testing of patient's bladder response to sacral neurostimulation by a temporary lead placed into S3 foramen followed by possible simultaneous implantation of the lead and IPG if the patient responded appropriately to the first step. Janknegt et al [7] first described the staged implantation approach in which an implanted S3 lead, rather than the temporary lead, was used for initial testing. The implanted S3 lead is externalized by an extension and stimulated by an external stimulator. The advantages of testing the patient in this manner include less chance of lead migration and better ability to predict long-term patient response because the implanted lead is chronically stimulated once the patient is deemed a test-responder. With the original InterStim technique, there is a chance that the patient's beneficial response to the temporary lead is not replicated when the S3 lead implantation step occurs because of the differences inherent in the temporary and permanent leads and the inability perfectly to replicate the lead position in the S3 foramen.

Current surgical approach to sacral neurostimulation

With the development of the minimally invasive percutaneous technique of S3 lead implantation, staged implantation has become widely

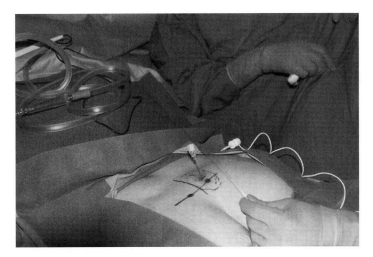

Fig. 1. The patient is in prone position and the camera is positioned on patient's left side. The patient has had a foramen needle inserted into the right S3 using cross-hair fluoroscopic technique (lines marked on back). The wire that is passed coaxially into the needle is also shown.

accepted. The usual approach for patients undergoing sacral neurostimulation is a first-stage procedure of percutaneous implantation of a tined lead into S3 foramen. After sacral neurostimulation through the implanted lead for anywhere between 1 to 4 weeks, if a patient has a significant improvement in bladder symptoms, then he or she undergoes implantation of an IPG during the second stage. If there is not a significant benefit, the implanted lead is removed and the IPG implant is not performed.

There is no consensus as to whether one or two implanted S3 leads should be performed as in the first stage. Bilateral implantation allows for testing for both the left and right S3 nerve roots. At the time of the second stage, the side that is less efficacious can be removed or remain implanted for possible backup in case the other side fails. Currently, there is no evidence that bilateral simultaneous stimulation has any added benefits to unilateral stimulation. Furthermore, there is not the ability to stimulate both wires with one IPG in the United States because the IPG is not a dual-channel stimulator. One needs to implant two IPGs for bilateral simultaneous stimulation. Nevertheless, bilateral implantation allows for

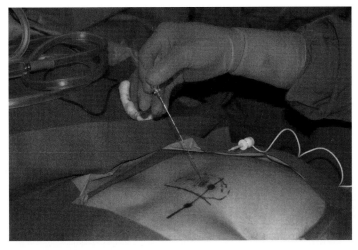

Fig. 2. The wire, which is part of the percutaneous lead introducer kit, has been passed through the needle to the level of the ventral S3 foramen using lateral fluoroscopic guidance. The needle was then moved back, leaving the wire in place.

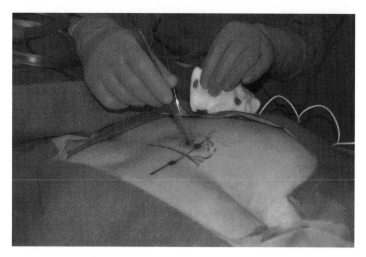

Fig. 3. Using a scalpel, a nick is made along the wire to facilitate passage of the introducer.

a more complete evaluation and possibly offers the patient a higher chance of responding to sacral neurostimulation.

Fig. 1 depicts a patient in prone position with a foramen needle in the right S3 foramen. The skin had been previously marked using fluoroscopy. The purple circles represent the expected locations of the S3 foramina. The reason that the foramen needle is inserted higher than the marked S3 site is because the needle has to be inserted at a 60-degree angle to the parallel rather than at 90 degrees to access the S3 foraminal canal. The wire from the introducer is shown being held by the left hand in the field. Once the foramen needle is in S3 and stimulation of the needle with an external stimulator by the cable (shown clipped to the drape in Fig. 1), the wire is placed through the needle and the needle is removed (Fig. 2) leaving the wire in place. A nick is made in the skin (Fig. 3) to allow for easier passage of the wider introducer. The introducer, with the obturator in place, is inserted coaxially down the wire (Fig. 4). Lateral fluoroscopy is required to determine the depth to insert the introducer. Because the tip of the obturator is metallic, it is visible on fluoroscopy. Furthermore, there is a radiopaque ring at the level of the tip of the plastic sheath of the introducer. The ring

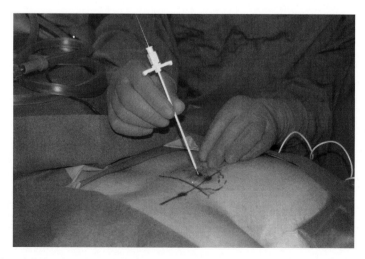

Fig. 4. The introducer is being passed coaxially down the wire so that the tip of the introducer lies just anterior to the ventral S3 foramen using lateral fluoroscopic guidance.

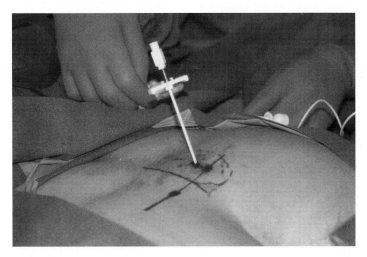

Fig. 5. The obturator within the introducer is now removed, while the sheath remains in position.

should be at the level of the ventral S3 foramen and the metal obturator just beyond the ventral S3 foramen. Once at the correct depth, the obturator is removed, leaving the sheath within the S3 foraminal canal (Fig. 5).

The tined lead, with four plastic collapsible projections, is inserted into the sheath under lateral fluoroscopic guidance (Fig. 6). The lead has four quadripolar contact points (Figs. 7, 8), which is not visible in Fig. 6 because it is already inside the sheath. The position for the lead is such that lead position #1 is straddling the ventral S3 foramen, meaning half of lead position #1 is anterior and the other half is posterior to the ventral sacral cortex (see Fig. 8). To test for proper motor and sensory responses in the patient, the sheath is moved back to a white line marked on the lead by the manufacturer to expose all quadripolar contact points, but without engaging the plastic projections (Fig. 9). Once stimulation confirms proper sensory and motor responses, the sheath is removed totally allowing the plastic projections to engage the soft tissues, anchoring the lead (Fig. 10). Note that in Fig. 10 another tined lead has been implanted into the left S3 foramen.

The next step is to bury the leads and to bring them out to a point where the future IPG may be implanted. In this particular patient, it was determined that a future IPG would be implanted in

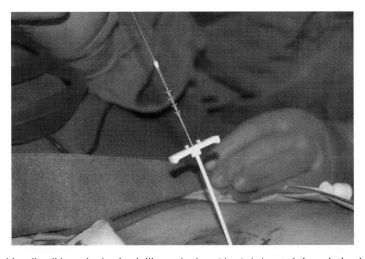

Fig. 6. The lead, with collapsible anchoring hook-like projections (tines), is inserted through the sheath into a proper position based on lateral fluoroscopy.

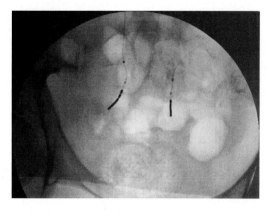

Fig. 7. Anteroposterior fluoroscopic view of the sacrum with two S3 tined leads at end of the case.

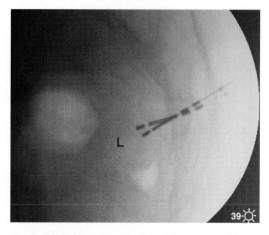

Fig. 8. Lateral fluoroscopic view of the sacrum with two S3 tined leads at end of the case.

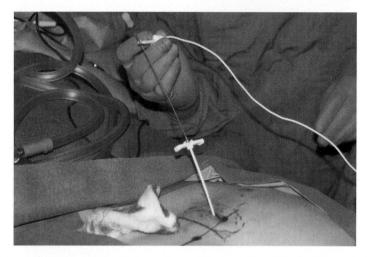

Fig. 9. The sheath is retracted to a set-point to expose the quadripolar leads within the S3 foraminal canal. The lead is connected to an external stimulator to ensure proper sensory and motor responses further to confirm proper positioning.

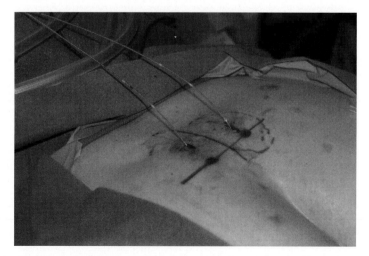

Fig. 10. Once the lead is confirmed to be in the correct position, the sheath is totally removed to engage the tines. A left S3 lead has also been percutaneously placed.

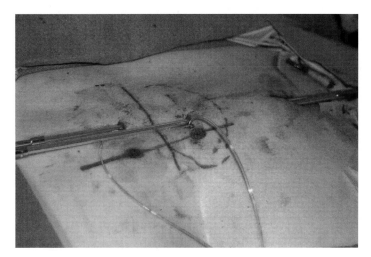

Fig. 11. Two tunnelers are placed from the right upper buttock area (site where future IPG will be located) to the lead insertion sites. The tunnelers contain trocars that are next removed, leaving the plastic sheaths in place. The free end of the leads are then passed through the sheaths so that they exit out the skin in the right upper buttock area.

the right upper buttock. A 2- to 3-cm transverse incision is made in the right upper buttock. Using a tunneler device supplied in a kit, the tunneler is passed from the exit point of the tined lead to the right upper buttock incision (Fig. 11). The trocar in the tunneler is removed leaving a plastic straw in position. The tined leads are then passed into the two straws so that they exit out the right upper buttock incision (Fig. 12). The leads are then connected to an external extension and connection site covered with a boot (see Fig. 12). The

external extensions are brought out superior to the right upper buttock incision using the tunneler device again (Fig. 13). This is to decrease risk of infection to the future IPG site at the right upper buttock. The excess length in the leads and the connection boots are buried in a subcutaneous pocket in the right upper buttock incision and this incision is closed with multilayered absorbable sutures (Fig. 14). The two small nicks over where the foramen needles were used to localize S3 are closed with simple interrupted absorbable sutures

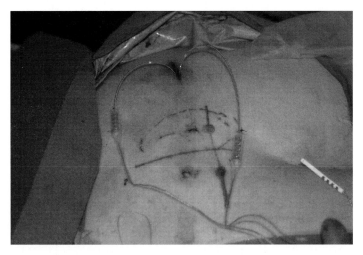

Fig. 12. The camera has moved position. The view is still from the patient's left side, but is more superior to the previous figures. This image shows the leads exiting from the right upper buttock. Also, the leads have been connected to external extensions and two boots cover this connection.

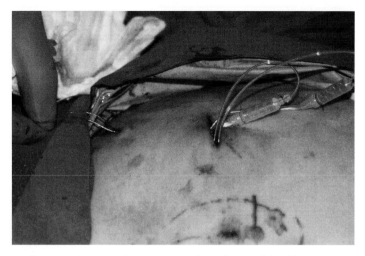

Fig. 13. Using the tunneler again, the external extensions are brought out of the skin at a separate site than the right upper buttock to prevent potential bacterial infection of the potential future IPG site. The two boots will be buried in the right upper buttock area.

(see Fig. 14). The exit site of the external extensions is dressed with dry gauze, but this site could be a conduit for bacteria and a distance separating this site from the right upper buttock incision where the future IPG sits is important to reduce chance of infections. Figs. 7 and 8 show the anteroposterior and lateral fluoroscopic images of the bilateral implanted leads.

Over the next 1 to 4 weeks, the patient is sequentially stimulated (one S3 at a time) by an external stimulator connected to the external extension to determine optimum bladder response. It is the opinion of the author that the maximum tolerable time be used to elicit maximum possible benefit of S3 neurostimulation. The lead on the side giving the best response is

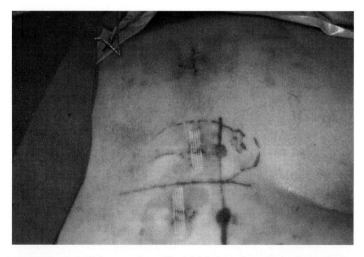

Fig. 14. This is an image at the end of the procedure. The initial sites where the leads were percutaneously placed are steri-stripped after closure with absorbable sutures. Underneath the right upper buttock incision site, which has also been closed with absorbable sutures, contains the two boots buried in a subcutaneous pocket. The external extensions are exiting the skin at a separate area from where the future IPG site will be located. The two leads can be marked with different colored sutures to differentiate the left from the right side.

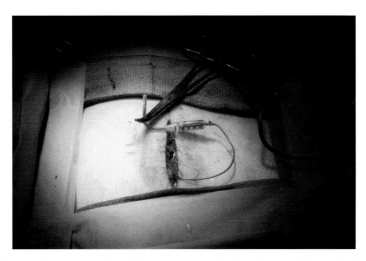

Fig. 15. This is the second stage procedure. The external extension has been cut (where the hemostat is) and the externalized portion discarded. The next step would be to disconnect the tined lead from the remnant of the external extension (bullet shaped area to the right of the hemostat). The tined lead is then connected to the IPG (not shown).

connected to the implanted IPG during the next second-stage surgery.

Fig. 15 depicts the first step of the second-stage IPG implantation. The right upper buttock incision is opened wider and the boots are exteriorized. The external extensions that remain sterile are cut and the booted connections are disconnected. At this point, the circulator nurse pulls out the external extensions and preserves the sterility of the surgical field. The tined lead that will be stimulated is connected to the IPG in the usual fashion. The other tined lead that will not be used can either be left alone and buried with the IPG into the right upper buttock or removed. To remove the tined lead, a small incision is made over the previous nick scar at the correct side. The lead is dissected out and pulled out with firm pressure. There is no need for fluoroscopy for the second stage.

Summary

Refinements in making surgical approaches in sacral neurostimulation less morbid and more efficient has resulted in this approach being a tenable option for those patients afflicted with idiopathic urinary urge incontinence, frequency-urgency syndrome, and nonobstructive urinary retention. Traditionally, these patients were relegated to suffering with their bladder symptoms because of the lack of options. Now, this form of

therapy, although not perfect, offers hope to many. Future refinements in treatment of these patients will be multifaceted including further improvements in surgical approaches, understanding pathophysiology, and better diagnostic tools.

References

[1] Schmidt RA, Senn E, Tanagho EA. Functional evaluation of sacral nerve root integrity: report of a technique. Urology 1990;35:388–92.

[2] Thon WF, Baskin LS, Jonas U, et al. Surgical principles of sacral foramen electrode implantation. World J Urol 1991;9:133–7.

[3] Chai TC, Mamo GJ. Modified techniques of S3 foramen localization and lead implantation in S3 neuromodulation Urology 2001;58:786–90.

[4] Hohenfellner M, Schultz-Lampel D, Dahms S, et al. Bilateral chronic sacral neuromodulation for treatment of lower urinary tract dysfunction. J Urol 1998;160:821–4.

[5] Scheepens WA, Weil EH, van Koeveringe GA, et al. Buttock placement of the implantable pulse generator: a new implantation technique for sacral neuromodulation. A multicenter study. Eur Urol 2001;40: 434–8.

[6] Spinelli M, Giardiello G, Gerber M, et al. New sacral neuromodulation lead for percutaneous implantation using local anesthesia: description and first experience. J Urol 2003;170:1905–7.

[7] Janknegt RA, Weil EHJ, Eerdmans PHA. Improving neuromodulation technique for refractory voiding dysfunctions: two-stage implant. Urol 1997;49: 358–62.

ELSEVIER
SAUNDERS

Urol Clin N Am 32 (2005) 37–40

UROLOGIC
CLINICS
of North America

Current Indications for Neuromodulation

Firouz Daneshgari, MD[a],*, M. Louis Moy, MD[b]

[a]Center for Female Pelvic Medicine and Reconstructive Surgery, Glickman Urological Institute, The Cleveland Clinic
Foundation, 9500 Euclid Avenue, Cleveland, OH 44195, USA
[b]Department of Urology, University of Pennsylvania, Penn Tower 9th Floor/4283, 300 South 33rd Street,
Philadelphia, PA 19104, USA

Neuromodulation is becoming part of the clinical armamentarium for treatment of a variety of lower urinary tract conditions. It increased usage stems from needs of patients who have exhausted all other therapeutic options. Currently, neuromodulation may consist of the use of nerve stimulation and injectable therapies. This article concentrates on nerve stimulation. Currently, there are two nerve stimulation modalities approved by the US Food and Drug Administration (FDA): sacral nerve stimulation (SNS; Interstim, Medtronic, Minneapolis, MN) and peripheral nerve stimulation (SANS).

Background

SNS involves stimulation of the sacral nerves to modulate the neural reflexes that influence the bladder, sphincter, and pelvic floor. The initial experience with SNS for use in bladder dysfunction was reported by Tanagho and Schmidt [1]. Since then, SNS using Interstim has been an invasive therapy approved by the FDA in 1997 for treatment of refractory urge incontinence. In April 1999, this approval was expanded to include significant urgency, frequency, and idiopathic urinary retention as indications for the use of SNS therapy. Worldwide, the number of implants has passed 15,000 in 2004, with more than 70% of the implants in the United States.

Reported outcomes and levels of evidence

Implantation of SNS consists of two steps. Stage one, or the trial stage, involves the placement of a stimulation lead next to the dorsal root of S3 for a test period between 1 and 4 weeks. If the patient's symptoms under the existing list of indications for SNS improve more than 50%, then the patient is a candidate to undergo stage 2 or the permanent step, in which the permanent neurostimulator is implanted in the soft tissue of the patient's buttock.

The reported outcomes of SNS usually include the response of patients to stage one (test stage) and to stage two (permanent implantation). Table 1 provides a summary of published reports of use of SNS.

No discussion on the assessment of treatment options is complete without a discussion on the issue of level of evidence. The evidence required in the medical literature is limited to data reported in clinical trials, specifically excluding expert opinion. This is similar to that required to determine the final judgment of a jury in a legal proceeding, which must be based on the material evidence presented during the trial. The judgment (opinion) of the jury is not evidence. Evidence is factual information presented.

International consultation on incontinence has adopted the Oxford level of evidence as the following categories:

Level 1. Usually involves meta-analysis of trials (randomized clinical trials or a good-quality randomized controlled trial or all-or-none studies in which "no treatment" is not an option (eg, vesicovaginal fistula).

Level 2. Includes low-quality randomized controlled trial or meta-analysis of good-quality

---

* Corresponding author.
E-mail address: daneshf@ccf.org (F. Daneshgari).

38 DANESHGARI & MOY

Table 1
Published reports of use of sacral nerve stimulation in various conditions of lower urinary tract dysfunction

Study	Total	Patients with UI			Patients with U/F		Patients with IUR		Follow-up
		Cured	>50%	Improved	>50%	Improved	>50%	Improved	
US National Patient Register	81		27/43		10/19		10/19		
Amundsen 2002	12		12/12	2/12					
Hedlund 2002	14		13/14	8/14					
Bosch 2000	45		27/45	18/45					
Shaker 1998	18		12/18	8/18					
Siegel 2000	112		21/41	19/41	16/29	5/29	29/42	24/42	
Schmidt 1999	34	16/34	10/34	26/34			16/34		18 mo
Grunewald 1999	39		13/18				18/21		
Jonas 2001	29						20/29		18 mo
Hassouna	25				14/25				12 mo
Aboseif 2002	32						18/20	2/20	24 mo

Abbreviations: IUR, idiopathic urinary retention; U/F, urgency frequency; UI, urge incontinence.

prospective cohort studies. These may include a single group when individuals who develop the condition are compared with others from within the original cohort group. There can be parallel cohorts, where those with the condition in the first group are compared with those in the second group.

Level 3. Evidence includes good-quality retrospective case-control studies where a group of patients who have a condition are matched appropriately (eg, for age, sex, and so forth) with control individuals who do not have the condition; and good-quality case series where a group of patients all with the same condition, disease, or therapeutic intervention are described without a comparison control group.

Level 4. Evidence includes expert opinion where the opinion is based not on evidence but on first principles (eg, physiologic or anatomic) bench research. The Delphi process can be used to give expert opinion or greater authority. In the Delphi process a series of questions are posed to a panel; the answers are collected into a series of options; the options are serially ranked; if a 75% agreement is reached then a Delphi consensus statement can be made.

Reports of clinical trials on urge incontinence, urgency frequency, and nonobstructive urinary retention

At this point in time SNS has been approved by the FDA for three indications: (1) urge

incontinence, (2) urgency frequency, and (3) nonobstructive urinary retention. SNS has also been reported to be used for other off-label indications, however, such as neurogenic bladders in multiple sclerosis, interstitial cystitis, and chronic pelvic pain. There are also reports regarding the possible benefits of bilateral SNS. Most of the reports on the nonformal usages of SNS appear in the form of abstracts or case series.

The initial report on the efficacy of SNS on treatment of refractory urinary urgent incontinence was reported in 1999 (level 2, because no placebo or sham control was used) [2]. This study reported the treatment of 76 patients with refractory urgent urinary incontinence from 16 contributing worldwide centers. The patients were randomized to immediate implantation and a control group with delayed implantation for a 6-month period. At 6 months, the number of daily incontinence episodes, severity of episodes, and absorbent pads or diapers replaced daily because of incontinence was significantly reduced in the stimulation group compared with the delayed group. Of the 34 stimulation group patients, 16 (47%) were completely dry, and an additional 10 (29%) demonstrated a greater than 50% reduction in incontinence episodes. The interesting finding was that during the therapy evaluation, the group returned to the baseline level of incontinence when the stimulation was inactivated. Complications were site pain of the stimulator implantation in 16%, implants infection in 19%, and leak migration in 7%.

The use of SNS in urgency frequency was reported in 2000 [3]. Similar to the previous design,

51 patients from 12 centers were randomized into an immediate stimulation group and a control group (25 and 26 patients, respectively) (level 2, because no placebo or sham control was used). Patients were followed for 1, 3, and 6 months, and afterward at 6-month intervals up to 2 years. At the 6-month evaluation, the stimulation group showed improvement in the number of voiding dailies (16.9 ± 9.7 to 9.3 ± 5.1); volume per void (118 ± 74 to 226 ± 124 mL); and degree of urgency (the rank 2.2 ± 0.6 to 1.6 ± 0.9). In addition, significant improvement in quality of life was demonstrated, as measured by SF-36.

The report of use of SNS in urinary retention was published in 2001 [4], and in this study 177 patients with urinary retention refractory to conservative therapy were enrolled from 13 worldwide centers between 1993 and 1998 (level 2, because no placebo or sham control was used). Thirty-seven patients were assigned to treatment and 31 to the control group. The follow-up was done at 1, 3, 6, 12, and 18 months. The treatment group showed 69% elimination of catheterization at 6 months and an additional 14% with greater than 50% reduction in catheter volume per catheterization. Temporary inactivation of SNS therapy resulted in significant increase in residual volume, but the effectiveness of central nervous stimulation was sustained for 18 months after implantation.

In 2000, a follow-up report of some of these patients was published (level 3) [5]. This report showed follow-up results after 3 years in all the improved indications. Fifty-nine percent of 41 patients had urinary urgent incontinence. Patients showed greater than 50% with 46% of patients being completely dry. After 2 years, 56% of the urgency frequency patients showed greater than 50% reduction in voids per day, and after 1 to 1.5 years, 70% of 42 retention patients showed greater than 50% reduction of catheter volume per catheterization. Other studies, generally case series, have published results of the use of SNS following its initial approval.

The results of the use of SNS in the United States population were published in 2002 (level 3) [6]. This publication showed the data collected from the United States patient registry. The report included the use of SNS in 81 patients with all three indications: 27 for urgent continence, 10 with urgency frequency, and 10 with urinary retention. In this report, 27 out of 43 patients with urgent continence, 10 out of 19 with urgency frequency, and 10 out of 19 with urinary retention showed improvement of more than 50%.

The results of an Italian registry were published in 2001 (level 3) [7]. This report included the reports of 196 patients (46 males and 150 females) for idiopathic urinary retention. Fifty percent of patients stopped catheterization and another 13% catheterized once a day at 1 year after implantation. At the 12-month follow-up, 50% of patients with hyperreflexia had less than one incontinence episode daily and the problem was completely solved in 66 patients. Of the patients with urgent continence, 39% were completely dry and 23% had less than one incontinence episode daily.

In Norway, the results of users of this modality were published in 2002 (level 3) [8]. The author reported the first 3 years of experience with 53 patients: 45 women and 8 men. This study showed similar results to previous studies.

Urinary retention

Aboseif et al [9] reported on the use of SNS in functional urinary retention (level 3). Thirty-two patients were evaluated and underwent temporary PNE. Those who had a least a 50% improvement in symptoms during the test period underwent permanent generator placement. All patients who went to permanent generator placement were able to void spontaneously. There were both an increase in voided volume (48 to 198 mL) and decrease in postvoid residual (315 to 60 mL). Eighteen of 20 patients reported a greater than 50% improvement in quality of life.

Peripheral nerve stimulation

Stoller et al [10] in 1987 reported that stimulation of the peripheral tibial nerve in pig-tailed monkeys was able to inhibit bladder instability (level 3). This initial work led to its use in patients with refractory overactive bladder. The Stoller afferent nerve stimulator (SANS) has been FDA-approved for use in refractory overactive bladder.

Method

A 34-gauge stainless steel needle is placed about 5 cm cephalad to the medial malleolus and the needle is advanced posterior to the tibia. Once in place the ground pad is placed on the calcaneus. A stimulator is then connected to the needle and the ground pad. With the stimulator on, flexion of the great toe indicates the correct needle position. Thirty-minute treatments then take place once a week for 10 to 12 weeks.

Results

Klinger et al [11] in 2000 performed a prospective trial on 15 patients with urgency-frequency syndrome. They underwent 12 stimulation with the SANS device (level 3). Ten patients responded with a reduction in voiding frequency per day (16 to 4) and daily leakage episodes (4 to 2.4). The only complication was one hematoma at the puncture site.

Govier et al [12] (level 3) in a multicenter study reported the efficacy of SANS in 53 patients. All patients had refractory OAB and were seen at five different sites in the United States. The patients completed a 12-week stimulation. Seventy-one percent of the patients had at least a 25% decrease in daytime or nighttime frequency. No adverse effects were noted.

Further readings

Bosch JL. Sacral neuromodulation: treatment success is not just a matter of optimal electrode position [review]. BJU Int 2000;85(Suppl 3):20–1.

Chartier-Kastler EJ, Ruud Bosch JH, Perrigot M, et al. Long-term results of sacral nerve stimulation (S3) for the treatment of neurogenic refractory urge incontinence related to detrusor hyperreflexia. J Urol 2000;164:1676–80.

Grunewald V, Hofner K, Thon WF, et al. Sacral electrical neuromodulation as an alternative treatment option for lower urinary tract dysfunction. Restor Neurol Neurosci 1999;14:189–93.

Janknegt RA, Hassouna MM, Siegel SW, et al. Long-term effectiveness of sacral nerve stimulation for refractory urge incontinence. Eur Urol 2001;39:101–6.

Shaker HS, Hassouna M. Sacral nerve root neuromodulation: an effective treatment for refractory urge incontinence. J Urol 1998;159:1516–9.

Shaker HS, Hassouna M. Sacral root neuromodulation in idiopathic nonobstructive chronic urinary retention. J Urol 1998;159:1476–8.

References

[1] Tanagho EA, Schmidt RA, Orvis BR. Neural stimulation for control of voiding dysfunction: a preliminary report in 22 patients with serious neuropathic voiding disorders. J Urol 1989;142:340.

[2] Schmidt RA, Jonas U, Oleson KA, et al. Sacral nerve stimulation for treatment of refractory urinary urge incontinence. Sacral Nerve Stimulation Study Group. J Urol 1999;162:352–7.

[3] Hassouna MM, Siegel S, Nyeholt AA, et al. Sacral neuromodulation in the treatment of urgency-frequency symptoms: A multicenter study on efficacy and safety. J Urol 2000;163(6):1849–54.

[4] Jonas U, Fowler CJ, Chancellor MB, et al. Efficacy of sacral nerve stimulation for urinary retention: results 18 months after implantation. J Urol 2001; 165:15–9.

[5] Siegel SW, Catanzaro F, Dijkema HE, et al. Long-term results of a multicenter study on sacral nerve stimulation for treatment of urinary urge incontinence, urgency-frequency, and retention. Urology 2000;56(6 Suppl 1):87–91.

[6] Pettit PD, Thompson JR, Chen AH. Sacral neuromodulation: new applications in the treatment of female pelvic floor dysfunction [review]. Curr Opin Obstet Gynecol 2002;14:521–5.

[7] Spinelli M, Bertapelle P, Cappellano F, et al. Chronic sacral neuromodulation in patients with lower urinary tract symptoms: results from a national register. J Urol 2001;166:541–5.

[8] Hedlund H, Schultz A, Talseth T, et al. Sacral neuromodulation in Norway: clinical experience of the first three years. Scand J Urol Nephrol Suppl 2002; 210:87–95.

[9] Aboseif K, Tamadon S, Chalfin S, et al. Sacral neuromodulation in functional urinary retention: an effective way to restore voiding. Br J Urol 2002;90: 662–5.

[10] Stoller M, Copeland S, Millard R, et al. The efficacy of acupuncture in reversing the unstable bladder in pig-tailed monkeys [abstract]. J Urol 1987;137:104A.

[11] Klinger H, Pycha A, Schmidbauer J, et al. Use of peripheral neuromodulation for treatment of detrusor overactivity: a urodynamic-based study. Urology 2000;56:766–71.

[12] Govier F, Litwiller S, Nitti V, et al. Percutaneous afferent neuromodulation for the refractory overactive bladder: results of a multicenter study. J Urol 2001;165:1193–8.

ELSEVIER
SAURDERS

Urol Clin N Am 32 (2005) 41–49

UROLOGIC
CLINICS
of North America

Canadian Experience in Sacral Neuromodulation

Mohamed Elkelini, MD,
Magdy M. Hassouna, MD, PhD, FRCSC, FACS*

*Division of Urology, Toronto Western Hospital, University Health Network, University of Toronto, 399 Bathurst Street,
MP 8-306, Toronto, Ontario M5T 2S8, Canada*

The function of the bladder is twofold: a reservoir to hold urine at low pressure and voiding to evacuate the urine. Disturbance of one or both of these functions results in urinary voiding dysfunction. The urinary bladder and outlet are under neural control from the sacral nerves. The latter are under influence from higher centers, particularly the pontine micturition center. The pontine micturition center receives neural input from the frontal lobe cortex, the cerebellum, and the basal nuclei, to mention a few. Any neurologic disturbances inflicted on one or more of these nerve structures result in voiding dysfunction secondary to neurogenic bladder. Voiding dysfunction can occur also in the absence of an overt neurologic lesion.

These patients suffer from different forms of incontinence, namely urge in conjunction with stress incontinence. Patients are also known to have pelvic floor dysfunction that results in lower urinary tract malfunction. Treatment of patients with conventional pharmacologic therapy does not achieve satisfactory results. Repeated surgical intervention aimed at denervating or augmenting the bladder is usually insufficient to control urge incontinence.

Sacral root neuromodulation is a relatively recent concept for the treatment of various voiding and storage dysfunctions, but is gaining wide acceptance among the international urology community. The principles were laid down by Tanagho and Schmidt [1,2] early in the 1980s. Since then, hundreds of patients have had neuroprostheses

implanted to treat various dysfunctions. Several reports have been published addressing different aspects. The indications have expanded, and now include urge incontinence and sensory urgency [3–5], idiopathic chronic urinary retention [4–8], pelvic pain [4–7], and interstitial cystitis [9].

Patients in any of the previously mentioned categories of bladder dysfunction undergo a screening test called percutaneous nerve evaluation (PNE), in which a temporary wire electrode is inserted in the S3 foramen. The patient is sent home with an external pulse generator for a few days. The patient records his or her voiding parameters in a voiding diary. Based on the latter, those patients who show 50% improvement in one or more of the voiding parameters are offered a permanent sacral foramen implanted electrode and an implantable pulse generator (IPG).

The current procedure used for PNE is the one described by Thon et al [7]. They used an angiocatheter with a finder needle to probe the foramen. The Canadian contribution was presented in the form of a spinal needle partly insulated. Currently, this needle was modified and supplied with the PNE kit from Medtronic (Minneapolis, MN). The angle recommended by the authors was 60 degrees to the skin. We reported a different technique. The main difference is in the angle of the probing needle. We used a 30- to 40-degree angle to the skin [10].

After the desirable response is obtained and the wire secured in place, the patient is sent home with the wire coupled to a portable pulse generator for a 5- to 7-day trial period of outpatient stimulation. Out of 50 patients tested by PNE for various voiding and storage problems, Elabbady et al [4] reported a satisfactory response to the subchronic testing in 17 patients. The response

Studies were supported by grants from the Canadian Institutes of Health Research and Medtronic (Minneapolis, MN).

* Corresponding author.
E-mail address: Magdy.Hassouna@uhn.on.ca
(M.M. Hassouna).

criteria in this study were rather strict, because only patients who showed more than 70% improvement in their main baseline symptoms were considered.

New Medtronic tined (3889) lead percutaneous implant

Tined leads offer sacral nerve stimulation (SNS) through a minimally invasive implant procedure. The use of local anesthesia allows for patient sensory response during the implant procedure. This response helps ensure optimal lead placement and may result in better patient outcomes. With previous lead designs, many physicians used general anesthesia, which did not allow for patient sensory response. Percutaneous lead placement allows the use of local anesthesia, which reduces the risks of general anesthesia and surgical incision. Furthermore, it may facilitate faster patient recovery time as a result of less muscle trauma and a minimized surgical incision. It also may reduce surgical time as a result of a sutureless anchoring procedure and reduced number of surgical steps (Figs. 1 and 2).

The Canadian experience with the tined lead was very favorable. It was shown that the lead did not show any migration of its original location as per radiographic findings.

The stages of percutaneous lead implant placement are as follows (Figs. 2–8):

1. The sacral foramen is located with a needle.

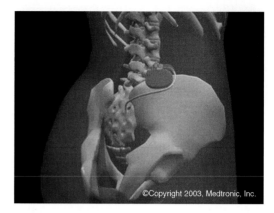

Fig. 2. Neurostimulator position after implantation.

2. A guidewire is fed through the needle.
3. The needle is removed and a metal-dilator is passed on top of the guidewire.
4. Under the guidance of fluoroscopy the end of the sheath is identified.
5. The metal-dilator is replaced with a plastic dilator.
6. The guidewire is removed.
7. The tined lead is fed through the plastic dilator.
8. There is stimulation of the lead to verify its position and produce the best motor and sensory responses.
9. The tined lead is deployed by removing the plastic dilator.
10. Stimulation of the tined lead throughout the procedure helps ensure proximity of the electrode to the sacral nerve.
11. The tined lead is fixed to fascia.

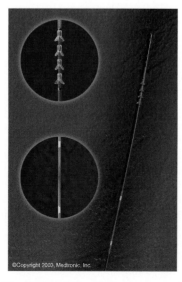

Fig. 1. New Medtronic tined lead percutaneous implant.

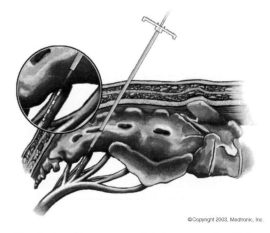

Fig. 3. Sacral foramen needle is inserted and guided to the desired location.

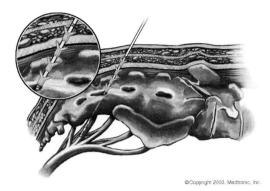

Fig. 4. Location is verified by electrical stimulation to the needle, and fluoroscopy is used to confirm the position of the needle in the S3 foramen.

Outcomes of the new tined lead

Spinelli et al [11] performed this new procedure on 32 patients. They reported that the success rate of this technique in selective patients for the permanent implant is significantly higher than what is reported in the literature. Beneficial clinical outcomes of the implanted patients confirm better patient selection with minimal complication.

This technique allows the possibility of more accurate patient selection by using the definitive lead for a longer test period before proceeding with the neurostimulator (IPG) implant.

University of Toronto experience

In the past few years, the authors' basic research has focused on the mechanism of bladder hyperreflexia after spinal cord injury. First, an

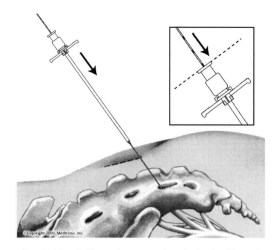

Fig. 6. Metal dilator is removed and plastic dilator is positioned.

animal model of spinal cord injury in rats was established by using female Sprague-Dawley rats; then urodynamics for the baseline and voiding dysfunction in controls and spinalized rats were studied. Afterward, VR1 expression was examined in dorsal root ganglia and bladder in controls and after spinal cord injury. Furthermore, the effects of neuromodulation of S1 roots on VR1 expression in rats after spinal cord injury were studied. The authors have demonstrated that neuromodulation can inhibit detrusor hyperreflexia and reduce neuropeptide content in dorsal root ganglia of rats with spinal cord injury [12]. Furthermore, neuromodulation of S1 nerve roots significantly reduced VR1 staining intensity in spinal cord

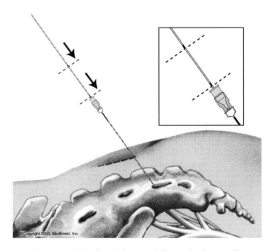

Fig. 5. Guidewire is inserted through the needle.

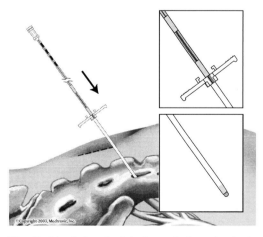

Fig. 7. Stimulation lead is inserted through plastic dilator.

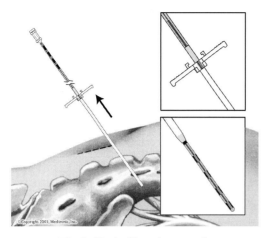

Fig. 8. Plastic dilator is removed.

injury rats, which indicates that neuromodulation can reduce VR1 expression in the spinal cord. The authors proposed that, at the molecular level, the underlying mechanism of neuromodulation could be the inhibition of VR1 expression in rats with spinal cord injury [13,14].

Another study was conducted to evaluate whether electrical stimulation has any adverse effect on pregnant rats and their fetuses. Electrical stimulation has been considered a contraindication in pregnant women with various voiding dysfunctions, because of the potential teratogenicity or abortion of the effect of electrical stimulation; however, whether electrical stimulation can cause abortion or fetal malformation is not known. The results of this study showed that electrical stimulation did not have any adverse effect on pregnant rats and their fetuses. Moreover, termination of pregnancy is not advised for prospective mothers when electrical stimulation has been performed inadvertently in early pregnancy [15].

Another contraindication for patients with an implanted bladder neurostimulator is to have an MR imaging examination. Eight MR imaging examinations at 1.5 T were conducted on six patients with an implanted bladder neurostimulator (InterStim neurostimulator, Medtronic, Minneapolis, MN). During the MR imaging session no patient showed symptoms that required stopping the examination. There was no change in perception of the stimulation according to patients' replies following reprogramming of the device. Devices were functioning properly, and no change in bladder functions was reported after MR imaging examinations. The authors propose that MR imaging can be safely done in patients

with implantable bladder neurostimulator provided that certain precautions are considered (unpublished data).

Results from a series of multicenter studies that the authors participated in have been recently published demonstrating the value of neuromodulation in the treatment of urgency-frequency symptoms [16], refractory urinary urge incontinence [17], and urinary retention [18]. In a retrospective study, the authors outlined the parameters of successful sacral root neuromodulation of the pelvic floor [19]. The following is a summary of the published data. In this study, a retrospective chart review was preformed on all patients who successfully underwent InterStim operations from 1993 to 2002 at the Toronto Western Hospital.

During this time period, 197 patients with voiding dysfunction (including urge incontinence, urgency-frequency, and chronic urinary retention) not responding to conventional therapy were seen in the clinic and underwent PNE as a screening test. Of these, 67 (34.01%) were successful and henceforth implanted with a neurostimulator on the third or fourth sacral nerve root. Fifty-eight were women and nine men, with ages ranging from 29 to 75 years old (average: 48.29).

Patients were followed-up after implantation for periods ranging from 3 months to 7 years. The implantable device used in 63 patients was the ITREL III (Medtronics, Minneapolis, MN). Four patients were implanted with the ITREL II. ITRELL III is the more recent model and allows for more versatility and patient control than previous models.

Screening test

All patients underwent PNE as a screening test. The steps of this test have been previously described [13,14]. Patients were asked to complete baseline-voiding diary before and during PNE, conducted for 3 to 7 days. The baseline-voiding diary is a standardized form of questions covering aspects of voiding function. The questions include frequency and voiding per day; voiding volume; number of pads used (in incontinent patients); degree of urgency; and the postvoid residual volume through self-catheterization in retention patients. A 50% improvement in baseline voiding symptoms during test stimulation is considered a cutoff value for the patient to qualify for surgical implantation of neuroprosthesis. All patients included in this study have achieved and maintained successful outcomes in one or more voiding parameters in the voiding diary. Implantation of the InterStim device was done under general anesthesia and involved the placement of a permanent electrode into the S3 foramen on one side through a small (5–7 cm) vertical incision over the sacrum.

Follow-up evaluations

Follow-up evaluations after implantation were done for each patient during visits at 1, 3, 6, 9, and 12 months after implantation, and every 6 months thereafter. In each visit the patient was requested to fill a voiding diary to document the efficacy of the therapy and side effects. The stimulation parameters were collected through an InterStim programmer (7432 Neurological Programmer, Medtronic).

Results

Results of the study are presented in Box 1.

The charge density provided by the present stimulator parameters was found to be in the safe zone. The configuration of electrode lead (model 3080, Medtronic) does not allow any local pressure on the nerve roots. The electrodes are located in proximity of the nerve root with minimal direct contact within the sacral foramina, causing minimal scarring of the nerve roots. The long-term effects show no evidence of neuronal damage.

Two reports have recently been published in the *Journal of Urology* concerning the authors' experience [5,8]. In the following section, the data are summarized.

Methodology

Inclusion and exclusion criteria

Patients with serious voiding dysfunction refractory to all conservative measures were included in the study. All underwent a detailed history and physical examination. The inclusion criteria were a diagnosis of either urgency-frequency or urge incontinence, or nonobstructive chronic urinary retention either complete or incomplete. Age was greater than 16 years. A normal upper urinary tract, adequate bladder volume (more than 100 mL), and no significant sphincteric pathology were essential prerequisites. Patients had to be willing and competent to complete the diaries and questionnaires of the study, and have the intention to comply with the study visit schedule.

Exclusion criteria included multiple sclerosis; Reiter's syndrome; severe uncontrolled diabetes mellitus or diabetes mellitus with peripheral neuropathy; pregnancy; anatomic limitations that prevent successful placement of an electrode, such as meningomyelocele; an active disease that limits the success of the procedure, such as active degenerative disk disease: spinal cord injury or cerebrovascular accident less than 6 months old; symptomatic urinary tract infection until treated: stress incontinence; pelvic pain not associated with voiding dysfunction or when it is the primary diagnosis; severe psychologic problems; and mechanical infravesical obstruction.

Study design

Patients who fit into the previously mentioned criteria underwent urodynamic study and were asked to complete two voiding diaries for four successive days each (baseline diaries). In addition, they completed Beck Depression Inventory and SF36 Quality of Life questionnaires.

After completion of these diaries the patients were subjected to PNE and sent home with a mobile pulse generator (Medtronics model 3625 screener) for subchronic testing. They were asked to complete another diary for four consecutive days (PNE diaries). A fourth diary was completed after the PNE once the symptoms returned baseline, and the baseline and the PNE diaries were compared. A 50% improvement of at least two major symptoms was chosen as a cutoff value in this study for the patient to qualify for implantation. After implantation, patients were followed up at 1, 3, and 6 months postimplantation, and every 6 months thereafter. Before each visit, a voiding diary and quality of life questionnaire were completed. During each visit, any complication was reported; stimulation parameters could be adjusted if necessary; and a free uroflowmetry was done, except at the 6-month visit when the patients underwent urodynamic studies instead. At this visit and after the urodynamics the implant was turned off and the patient instructed to complete a diary after returning to the baseline. After completion of the diary the implant was turned on again [5,8].

Results

Results of the peripheral nerve evaluation

One hundred and four patients with various serious voiding dysfunctions underwent PNE to

---

Box 1. Results of parameters of successful sacral root neuromodulation study

Amplitude
Amplitude (V) average: 1.462
Amplitude (V) upper limit average: 5.007
Amplitude (V) lower limit average: 0.3
The amplitude of stimulation in 67 patients ranged between 0.2 and 6.8 V. The average was
    1.462 V.

Pulse width (millisecond)
Pulse width (millisecond) average: 204.090 µs.
The pulse width ranged between 120 and 270 µs. Most patients (58) had a 210 µs pulse
    width. This is based on patient comfort level.

Rate (pulse per second)
Rate (pulse per second) average: 9.018
The pulse rate ranged from 2 to 20 pulses per second. Most patients (49) had a pulse rate of
    10 pulses per second. This is also based on patient tolerance and comfort level.

Mode (cycling versus continuous)
Sixty-one patients had cycling mode (91%), whereas only six patients (9%) were in
    continuous mode. Cyclic mode has the benefit of maintaining the patient's sense of
    awareness of the pelvic floor. Sixty-one patients had cycling mode of stimulation for 10
    seconds on and 5 seconds off. The stimulation cycle starts at 2 seconds ramping.

On time (seconds)
On time (seconds) average: 12.243.

Off time (seconds)
Off time (seconds) average: 4.765

Electrode assignment
All patients except one had the stimulator in monopolar fashion, with the case of IPG being
    positive. The active electrodes were arranged mainly between the distal two (see Fig. 1).

Electrode laterality and position
Most electrodes were placed in the third right sacral foramina and the third left sacral
    foramina. One patient had stimulation in both foramina, and three patients underwent the
    new tined lead sacral stimulation.

Load impedance
The load impedance was found to range from 578 to 1537 Ω (W). None of the patients had an
    impedance of more than 2000 W.

Change in amplitude over time
The patients were able to increase the amplitude to ensure proper perception of stimulation
    in the perineal area. There was a gradual increase in amplitude starting from 6 months
    until 36 months, with this increase getting significantly larger after that.

---

determine their responsiveness to neuromodula-tion. Physical examination disclosed no abnor-mality except tenderness or inability to control the pelvic floor, demonstrated in an inability to relax or contract the levator ani on command. Upper tract imaging and cystoscopy did not show abnormalities. These patients had failed all other conservative measures and procedures to treat their condition, including pharmacotherapy in the form of antispasmodics, anticholinergics, antide-pressants, smooth and skeletal muscle relaxants, α-blockers, and antibiotics to treat associated urinary tract infection. In most of the cases several courses of different medications had been tried. In addition, other pharmacotherapeutic agents were instilled in the bladder, such as heparin, dimethyl sulfoxide, and chiorpactin. Apart from the pharmacotherapy, a wide variety of surgical procedures were of no benefit to these patients. This included urethral dilatation, bladder neck resection or incision, bladder neck suspension or sling procedure, and enterocystoplasty. The direct causative agent in these patients was not always clear. Pelvic or perineal trauma, in the form of hysterectomy episiotomy, dilatation and curettage, and sexual abuse, was the most common single agent that preceded the occurrence of the symptoms, especially in the retention group.

Forty-one of these patients showed a significant improvement in their voiding diary parameters and qualified for a permanent neuroprosthetic implant: 20 of these were in the urgency-frequency or urge incontinence group (urge group), and 21 were in the retention group. Thirty-eight of the qualified patients have been implanted and three are still awaiting implantation. The remaining patients did not show an adequate response to PNE and hence did not qualify for a permanent neuroprosthesis.

It was noticeable that all the changes in diary parameters observed during PNE in the good responders persisted after implantation with no significant difference. There was no statistically significant difference between data obtained with PNE and those obtained at any point during follow-up in patients qualified for implantation. All patients returned to their baseline status after completion of the PNE, although in some this took a few days to occur.

Results of the urge group

Eighteen patients with urge incontinence who showed a significant improvement in response to PNE have been given a sacral root implant (Medtronics ITREL I, II, or Interstim). The mean age at the time of presentation was 42.3 ± 3.3 (22–67) years and the duration of the urinary symptoms was 6.6 ± 1.3 (1.2–18.8) years. All patients except two were women. The average follow-up duration in this group was 18.8 (3–83) months [5].

Sacral root neuromodulation effectively improved incontinence in this group of patients. This was reflected in many aspects. The average number of incontinence episodes per 24 hours decreased significantly after implantation and remained statistically lower than pretreatment for as long as the patients were followed-up. This was also demonstrated when the data were analyzed on an individual basis. Eight patients became completely dry after the surgery, and four had average leakage episodes of one or less daily. In fact, all patients except one showed either cure or improvement. Furthermore, urinary urgency and sense of emptying improved significantly. Associated pelvic pain decreased significantly [5]. Eight patients had associated chronic retention. The improvement of their voiding behavior was similar to that of the retention group, which is discussed in the following section [5].

The clinical improvement was associated with improvement in the urodynamic data. Voided volumes during the uroflowmetry increased up to twofold when comparing the baseline with the postoperative follow-up. Peak and mean flow rate stayed within the preoperative normal ranges. Cystometrogram showed the disappearance of bladder instability in only one of the four patients who showed it preoperatively. In the other three the bladder volume at which these contractions occurred increased from 80 to 124 mL. Bladder volume at first sensation increased by 50% from 133.17 ± 25.31 mL preoperative to 203.75 ± 42.29 mL 6 months postimplant. Cystometric bladder capacity increased by 15% from 291.93 ± 48.32 to 335.83 ± 51.05 mL. Pressure-flow studies in the patients with pure urge incontinence, as expected, demonstrated no difference [5]. Patients who completed 18-month follow-up in both groups (urge and retention) showed that their initial improvement in symptomatology persisted in the long term [5].

The amplitude of the stimulating current needed to be increased within the first 4 weeks and stabilized thereafter. Although variable from one patient to another, the current amplitude was in the 2-V range, with a pulse width of 210 μs and frequency of 2 to 15 Hz in most patients [5].

Analysis of the Beck Depression Index and the Quality of Life questionnaires showed some improvement, which was progressive in most of the items. This improvement ranged from 10% to 40% [5].

Results of the retention group

Twenty patients with idiopathic nonobstructive chronic urinary retention have been implanted to date. All but one were women. The average age of presentation was 33.67 ± 2.2 (19.43–55.66) years. The average duration of urinary retention at the time of presentation was

5.23 ± 1.1 (1.17–19) years. The mean follow-up was 15.17 (1–74) months. Two patients were lost to follow-up and their data were not included in the study. All patients were dependent on clean intermittent catherization (CIC) at the time of presentation [8].

There was a significant improvement in both the voided volumes and residual urine. The percentage of the residual urine to total urinary output dropped from 78.3% to 5.5% to 10.2% in the postoperative follow-up visits. Associated pelvic pain also demonstrated a significant improvement. All patients reported a subjective improvement in all their symptoms, including their sensation of emptiness after voiding. There was also an impressive decrease in the urinary tract infection rate after implantation [8].

The clinical improvements were translated to urodynamic data. Voided volumes, peak and mean flow rates, and residual volumes were almost normalized. No significant difference was shown in the data of the cystometrogram. Pressure-flow studies after implantation were within normal values [8].

Complications

None of the complications encountered was major or life-threatening: in fact, most were within expectations. The most important and frequent complication of PNE is wire migration before the end of the 4-day testing period. Regarding the permanent implant procedure the complications included superficial wound infection in two patients, and implant failure in one patient necessitating replacement of the IPG. Erosion of the extension cable toward the skin in two patients was corrected by burying the wire under the skin. Electrode migration in two patients required exploration and repositioning. Pain at the site of the implant required change of site in one patient, and there was persistent back pain radiating to the lower limbs in two patients for several weeks after surgery. None of these complications was irreversible and did not result in any nerve damage. Four implants had to be replaced for battery failure after 4 to 6 years of use [5,8].

Summary

The application of sacral nerve modulation and stimulation has gained wide acceptance as a tool to enhance the control of voiding. The simplicity of the technique has made the therapy appealing for refractory cases of voiding dysfunction. The percutaneous screening test is mandatory for the success of the therapy. Long-term follow-ups have shown efficacy and safety in patients with voiding dysfunction.

Sacral nerve modulation is an effective modality in the treatment of various voiding and storage dysfunction. The tined lead offers a minimally invasive implant procedure. The simplicity of the procedure and the patient's sensory awareness help to ensure best lead placement. Furthermore, local anesthesia instead of general anesthesia allows faster patient recovery and reduces complications. Finally, sacral neuromodulation offers a modality in the management of patients with voiding dysfunction.

References

[1] Schmidt RA. Applications of neurostimulation. Urol Neurourol Urodyn 1988;7:585.
[2] Tanagho EA, Schmidt RA. Electrical stimulation the management of neurogenic bladder. J Urol 1988;l40:1331.
[3] Bosch J, Groen J. Sacral (S3) segmental nerve stimulation as a treatment for urge incontinence in patients with detrusor instability: results or chronic electrical stimulation using an implantable neural prosthesis. J Urol 1995;154:504.
[4] Elabbady AA, Hassouna MM, Elhilali MM. Neural stimulation for chronic voiding dysfunctions. J Urol 1994;152:2076.
[5] Shaker HS, Hassouna M. Sacral nerve root neuromodulation: effective treatment for refractory urge incontinence. J Urol 1998;159:1516–9.
[6] Vapnek TM, Schmidt RA. Restoration of voiding in chronic urinary retention using neuroprosthesis. World J Urol 1991;9:142.
[7] Thon WF, Baskin LS, Jonas U, et al. Neuromodulation of voiding dysfunction and pelvic pain. World J Urol 1991;9:138.
[8] Shaker HS, Hassouna M. Sacral root neuromodulation in idiopathic nonobstructive chronic urinary retention. J Urol 1998;159:1476–8.
[9] Fall M. Conservative management of chronic interstitial cystitis: transcutaneous electrical nerve stimulation and transurethral resection. J Urol 1985;133:774.
[10] Hassouna MM, Elhilali MM. Role of the sacral root stimulator in voiding dysfunctions. World J Urol 1991;9:145.
[11] Spinelli SI, Giardiello C, Arduini A, et al. New percutaneous technique of sacral nerve stimulation has high initial success rate: preliminary results. Eur Urol 2003;43:70–4.

[12] Shaker HS, Wang Y, Loung D, et al. Role of c-afferent fibers in the mechanism of action of sacral nerve root neuromodulation in chronic spinal cord injury. Br J Urol 2000;85:905.

[13] Zhou Y, Wang Y, Abdelhady M, et al. Change of vanilloid receptor 1 following neuromodulation in rats with spinal cord injury. J Surg Res 2002;107:140–4.

[14] Zavara P, Sahi S, Hassouna MM, et al. An animal model for the neuromodulation of neurogenic bladder dysfunction. Br J Urol 1998;82:267–71.

[15] Wang Y, Hassouna MM. Electrical stimulation has no adverse effect on pregnant rats and fetuses. J Urol 1999;162:1785–7.

[16] Siegel S, Catanzaro F, Dijkema H, et al. Sacral neuromodulation in the treatment of urgency-frequency symptoms: a multicenter study on efficacy and safety. J Urol 2000;163:1849–54.

[17] Schmidt RA, Jonas U, Oleson KA, et al. Sacral nerve stimulation for treatment of refractory urge incontinence. J Urol 1999;162:352–7.

[18] Jonas U, Fowler CJ, Chancellor MB, et al. Efficacy of sacral nerve stimulation for urinary retention: results 18 months after implantation. J Urol 2001;165:15–9.

[19] Bin Mahfooz A, Elmayergi N, Abdelhady M, et al. Parameters of successful sacral root neuromodulation of the pelvic floor: a retrospective study. Can J Urol 2004;11:1749–54.

**ELSEVIER
SAUNDERS**

Urol Clin N Am 32 (2005) 51–57

**UROLOGIC
CLINICS
of North America**

European Experience with Bilateral Sacral Neuromodulation in Patients with Chronic Lower Urinary Tract Dysfunction

Ph. E.V. van Kerrebroeck, MD, PhD[a],*, W.A. Scheepens, MD, PhD[a],
R.A. de Bie, MD, PhD[b], E.H.J. Weil, MD, PhD[a]

[a]Department of Urology, Maastricht University Hospital, P. Debyelaan 25, PO Box 5800, 6202 AZ,
Maastricht, The Netherlands
[b]Department of Epidemiology, Maastricht University Hospital, P. Debyelaan 25, PO Box 5800, 6202 AZ,
Maastricht, The Netherlands

Unilateral sacral nerve stimulation (SNS) using the technique described by Tanagho and Schmidt [1] is a relatively new treatment modality for patients who have various refractory voiding dysfunctions. The classical unilateral technique consists of an electrode fixed in the S3 foramen and connected to an implanted pulse generator. The effectiveness of unilateral SNS has been reported in various clinical trials for the treatment of urgency/frequency, urge incontinence, and idiopathic urinary retention [2–4]. Patients who experience a sufficient subjective and objective improvement during a percutaneous nerve evaluation test are selected for final implant of a neuromodulation system [5,6].

Although temporary and chronic SNS can result in impressive clinical improvement up to complete relief of symptoms, many patients improve only partially, requiring further pad use or intermittent catheterization [2,4,7,8]. With this initial technique, follow-up results obtained 18 months after unilateral stimulation showed a clinical benefit in 76% of urge-incontinent patients and in 71% of patients who had urinary retention. Several methods have been developed in order to improve further these results.

Percutaneous test stimulation is the only method available to evaluate whether neuromodulation leads to a significant improvement in an individual [9]. This method also closely resembles implantation of the unilateral sacral neuromodulation system. A new test lead design allowed for better identification of candidates for sacral neuromodulation and reduced the chances of lead migration [10,11]. Bilateral sacral neuromodulation has been suggested as a more effective technique for voiding dysfunction in animal studies [12], as well as in neurologically intact patients [13].

Scientific basis of bilateral stimulation

Schultz-Lampel and Lindstrom [12,14] performed neurophysiologic studies to compare the efficacy of unilateral and bilateral SNS and to find a scientific basis for the application of bilateral neurostimulation in the clinical setting. In their experiments they reproduced clinical sacral foramen stimulation in isolated S2 SNS in choralose-anaesthetised cats.

A comparison was made between unilateral left and right stimulation and bilateral S2 stimulation. Isolated SNS had excitatory and inhibitory effects on the bladder and both effects depended consistently on stimulation frequency and intensity. Bladder excitation and inhibition were considered as reflex responses because they were abolished after transection of the dorsal roots.

* Corresponding author.
 E-mail address: Kerrebroeck@urology.azm.nl (Ph.E. V. van Kerrebroeck).

In all experiments, bladder excitation occurred at $0.8\times$ to $1.0\times$ threshold of alpha motor axons with a maximum at $1.2\times$ threshold. At $1.0\times$ to $1.2\times$ threshold, bladder inhibition occurred after cessation of stimulation, whereas bladder inhibition during stimulation started at $1.4\times$ threshold and increased with increasing intensities. Bilateral stimulation at the same segmental level induced effective bladder inhibition even at subthreshold intensities ($0.8-1.0\times$). Compared with unilateral stimulation, bilateral stimulation did not increase the excitatory response but did cause a significant increase in bladder inhibition (decrease of bladder pressure in $33\% \pm 4\%$).

These experiments indicate that bilateral stimulation at the same level produced a pronounced summation effect of two unilateral stimulations. In contrast, however, simultaneous stimulation of several ipsilateral segments at different levels (eg, S2 and S3 at one side) did not increase bladder inhibition.

Based on these animal experiments, one may conclude that in terms of bladder inhibition, unilateral sacral neuromodulation can be applied only at suboptimal stimulation parameters because uncomfortable skeletal muscle contractions limit stimulation at optimal inhibitory intensities. Bilateral SNS, however, can achieve effective bladder inhibition at intensities below the muscle-twitch threshold without producing problematic side effects. The authors concluded that potentially bilateral sacral neuromodulation may be more effective at lower stimulation intensities, thus reducing unhelpful side effects and potential nerve damage, and possibly increasing the life of the stimulator battery.

Clinical application of bilateral stimulation

Even before the results of research on bilateral sacral nerve neuromodulation were published, some clinicians, especially in Germany, used bilateral neuromodulation in the clinical setting [13,15]. The basis for clinical application was the bilateral innervation of the bladder [16–18]. In this clinical trial, however, the authors not only used bilateral stimulation, but the position and the design of the electrode were altered to increase the stimulation efficacy by rendering the electrode–nerve interaction more precise and confining the stimulation current to the target nerve. To do so, a small sacral laminectomy was performed and electrodes were placed in direct contact with the

nerve. The authors describe 17 patients implanted since 1994. With a follow-up between 9 and 28 months in the first 11 patients, a success rate of 50% for complete relief of symptoms is cited. In the second series of six patients with a follow-up of 13.6 months (3–22 months), one failure is encountered. These results are obtained, however, with some complications, requiring removal of the implant in two patients.

These authors claim that the clinical results of bilateral stimulation showed an increased efficacy. No direct comparison between unilateral and bilateral was made, however, and different electrodes were used compared with the unilateral technique, including a different surgical approach. Moreover, no published long-term follow-up data are available on these patients.

The only study published comparing the unilateral approach with the bilateral approach is a prospective, randomized, crossover trial, in which each patient underwent unilateral as well as bilateral test stimulation to assess the possible advantages of bilateral stimulation [19].

This study included 33 patients who had chronic voiding dysfunction, defined as urge incontinence with or without urodynamic instabilities, complete urinary retention, and incomplete voiding with residual of more than 100 mL. The patients were randomized in a two-arm crossover design (Fig. 1) after signed informed consent. This design was used so patients could act as their own control group; therefore, it required a smaller sample size.

All 33 patients subsequently underwent a bilateral trial test stimulation of the sacral nerves in a standardized manner [4,5]. The test lead was connected to an external stimulation device suitable for bilateral stimulation (Dualscreen 3628, Medtronic, Minneapolis, Minnesota). This stimulator delivers alternating pulses left and right, as in the case of bilateral implant with the synergy implantable pulse generator (Medtronic Synergy 7427, Medtronic Europe, Tolochenaz, Switzerland). Left and right amplitudes can be programmed individually, and were programmed at an amplitude just above sensory threshold. Patients were instructed to adjust the stimulation amplitude if necessary. Therefore, patients could not be blinded for unilateral or bilateral stimulation.

Unilateral and bilateral test stimulation was continued for at least 72 hours. Patients were assigned randomly to start with either bilateral or unilateral stimulation. Between the stimulation

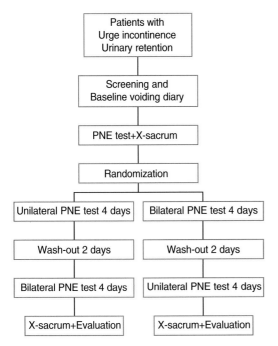

Fig 1. Flowchart of percutaneous nerve evaluation (PNE) test, interrupted by 2-day washout period. Diaries were completed during all phases and at baseline voiding. After implantation of leads and at end of 10-day test, anterior or posterior and lateral sacral radiographs (x-sacrum) were obtained.

episodes a 2-day washout interval of at least 48 hours was scheduled. During this period the external stimulator was switched off, so no stimulation was applied to the nerves. After this interval patients crossed over to unilateral or bilateral stimulation, respectively. The unilateral side (left or right) was chosen based on where the best response at the lowest amplitude was necessary to elicit the proper sensory response during acute testing. No contralateral testing was used because the test stimulation protocol would last an additional 4 days of stimulation plus an additional 2-day washout period, which would increase chances of lead migration and infection. In addition, during normal unilateral percutaneous nerve evaluation testing, normally the side with the best response using the lowest amplitude also was chosen for evaluation.

Standardized voiding diaries were used to record voiding, catheterization, and leaking episodes [2,3]. The voiding diaries were completed at baseline and during the unilateral and bilateral stimulation periods and washout period.

Anterior or posterior and lateral sacral radiographs were taken after implantation of the temporary lead and at the end of the test stimulation period to confirm lead positioning or possible migration. After 10 days the temporary leads were removed and voiding diaries were analyzed (see Fig. 1).

If lead migration occurred during the test, proven by sacral radiograph and loss of appropriate reactions, the patient was excluded from study because no true bilateral treatment effect could be expected. A difference of 50% between unilateral and bilateral stimulation was assumed to be clinically relevant and worth the effort and costs for bilateral stimulation, as is the case of unilateral stimulation. A power analysis (Pocock) showed that 12 patients were needed to show 50% difference between unilateral and bilateral stimulation ($\alpha 0.05$–1-β 80%).

For analysis, the voiding results were stratified for urge incontinence and urinary retention (patients who had voiding difficulty and complete urinary retention). Based on the voiding diary data and questionnaire information, comparative analyses of baseline to unilateral, baseline to bilateral, and unilateral to bilateral, respectively, were performed using the Wilcoxon signed ranks test with $P < 0.05$ considered statistically significant. SPSS software 9.0 (SPSS, Chicago, Illinois) was used for all data analysis.

The first postpercutaneous nerve evaluation radiographs showed that the electrodes were situated through the foramen of S3 in 31 patients and through S4 in two patients. Through randomization 16 of the 33 patients started with unilateral stimulation and 17 started with bilateral stimulation. The postpercutaneous nerve evaluation sacral radiographs at the end of the last stimulation period revealed unilateral lead migration in eight patients, and the appropriate reactions also were lost. Therefore, 12 patients who had urge incontinence and 13 who had retention were analyzed.

The urge incontinence group had a significant reduction in pad use compared with baseline to unilateral and bilateral stimulation. No significant difference was found between unilateral and bilateral stimulation. The severity of leakage reduced significantly compared with baseline to stimulation with no significant difference between the groups. A significant reduction also was seen in the number of voids per 24 hours compared with baseline, with no significant difference between the groups. Finally, a significant increase in

54   VAN KERREBROECK et al

volume per void was found, with no significant difference between groups (Fig. 2).

In the retention group the volume per void did not increase significantly during unilateral stimulation, but did increase significantly during bilateral stimulation. Comparing the volume per void between unilateral and bilateral stimulation, no significant difference was found during bilateral stimulation. The most important factor in

these patients was catheterized volume, which decreased significantly from baseline with no significant difference between groups (see Fig. 2).

The questionnaires revealed no significant subjective difference between the unilateral and bilateral stimulation period, in the urge incontinence ($P = 0.541$) or retention ($P = 0.362$) groups. Two patients with retention, however, started voiding only during bilateral stimulation with residuals of

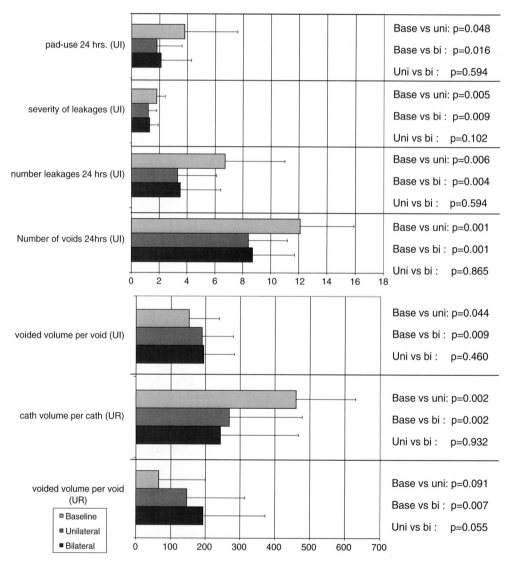

Fig. 2. Key voiding diary data of urge incontinent (UI) and urinary retention (UR) groups at baseline and during unilateral (uni) and bilateral (bi) stimulation. Significance levels compare baseline versus unilateral stimulation (base vs uni), baseline versus bilateral stimulation (base vs bi), and unilateral versus bilateral (uni vs bi). Severity of leakages is quantified as 0, no leakage; 1, drops of urine loss; 2, 3–8 mL urine loss; and 3, totally wet pad or diaper. Volumes are presented in mL. Cath volume per cath, catheterized volume per catheterization.

less than 100 mL. Both patients underwent a bilateral implant with the implantable pulse generator (Medtronic Synergy 7427) and still are voiding with less than 100 mL residual urine after 6 months of follow-up (Fig. 3), during which both patients completed a voiding diary for at least 72 hours. They performed clean intermittent self-catheterization at least once daily for retention measurements and no longer perform catheterization.

Discussion

Innervation of the bladder is considered bilateral, because each half of the bladder has its own confined innervation [16–18]. The small bladder afferents (Aδ and C fibers) are conducting the sensations of noxious stimuli, urge, and bladder distention [18], and also are considered bilateral through the pelvic nerve. Therefore, unilateral neuromodulation might be only partially effective, either by not influencing the entire bladder or allowing new formation of pathophysiologic pathways. Consequently, bilateral neuromodulation was introduced and has been propagated as a more effective method of sacral neuromodulation [20,21].

In a cat animal model, bilateral neuromodulation was more effective in inhibiting detrusor contractions than unilateral or multisegmental (multiple ipsilateral sacral nerves) neuromodulation [12].

Bilateral stimulation of the S3 nerve also has been reported as a tool to treat stress incontinence in patients who have spinal cord injury after implantation of a sacral anterior root stimulator and posterior rhizotomies [21,22]. A high amount of current is necessary to achieve constant contraction of the pelvic floor, however. These reports suggest that bilateral sacral neuromodulation is a better method for neuromodulation of the lower urinary tract. No comparison with the unilateral method has been performed in a clinical setting, however.

Recent data do not support the effectiveness of bilateral implantation for most patients. In a series of 25 patients there was no additional effect of bilateral compared with unilateral stimulation in 23 patients. Only two patients (8%) had additional benefit during bilateral compared with unilateral stimulation. These two patients, who had complete urinary retention, started voiding to completion only during bilateral stimulation. The reason could be that with bilateral stimulation sufficient sacral nerve afferents are stimulated to achieve marked effect at the level of the central nervous

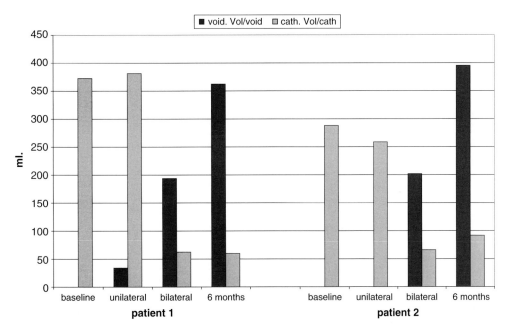

Fig. 3. Diary data of voided volume per void (void. Vol/void) and catheterized volume per catheterization (cath. Vol/cath) of two patients who started voiding only during bilateral stimulation. Both were implanted with implantable pulse generator and are still voiding with less than 100 mL residual urine after 6 months of follow-up.

system. All other patients who had urinary retention had no additional benefit from bilateral stimulation. No factor could be found to predict possible suitable candidates for bilateral stimulation other than urinary retention. It is possible that in these patients only bilateral neuromodulation provides sufficient electrical input to the sacral nerves to achieve a clinical effect. In both patients with retention the Synergy implantable pulse generator was used for bilateral stimulation, and after 6 months of follow-up, both are voiding with less than 100 mL residual urine (see Fig. 3).

Thus, some individuals may benefit from bilateral neuromodulation. During unilateral stimulation, however, 92% of patients achieved more than sufficient improvement of complaints; therefore, bilateral stimulation could not produce additional results. In terms of cost-effectiveness, however, unilateral should be tried before bilateral sacral neuromodulation. If a unilateral percutaneous nerve evaluation test fails, a bilateral test should be considered. If a bilateral test is successful, patients can be implanted with the bilateral neuromodulation system.

Summary

Although there is experimental and clinical evidence that bilateral stimulation of the sacral nerves could lead to summation effects, no significant differences in unilateral versus bilateral neuromodulation could be demonstrated in a comparative trial. In some individuals, however, only bilateral stimulation relieved symptoms. Therefore, if a unilateral percutaneous nerve evaluation test fails, a bilateral test should be considered. Further clinical research with long-term follow-up will allow the identification of which patients could benefit from bilateral stimulation with greater specificity and ameliorate further the long-term results achieved with unilateral SNS.

References

[1] Tanagho EA, Schmidt RA. Electrical stimulation in the clinical management of the neurogenic bladder. J Urol 1988;140:1331–9.

[2] Hassouna MM, Siegel SW, Lycklama à Nyeholt AA, et al. Sacral neuromodulation in the treatment of urgency-frequency symptoms: a multicenter study on efficacy and safety. J Urol 2000;163:1849–54.

[3] Schmidt R, Jonas U, Oleson K, et al. Sacral nerve stimulation for treatment of refractory urinary urge incontinence. Sacral Nerve Stimulation Study Group. J Urol 1999;162:352–7.

[4] Jonas U, Fowler CJ, Chancellor MB, et al. Efficacy of sacral nerve stimulation for urinary retention: results 18 months after implantation. J Urol 2001; 165:15–9.

[5] Schmidt R, Senn E, Tanagho E. Functional evaluation of sacral nerve root integrity. Report of a technique. Urology 1990;35:388–92.

[6] Siegel S. Management of voiding dysfunction with an implantable neuroprosthesis. Urol Clin North Am 1992;19:163–70.

[7] Bosch JL, Groen J. Sacral nerve neuromodulation in the treatment of patients with refractory motor urge incontinence: long-term results of a prospective longitudinal study. J Urol 2000;163:1219–22.

[8] Weil E, Ruiz Cerda J, Eerdmans P, et al. Sacral root neuromodulation in the treatment of refractory urinary urge incontinence: a prospective randomized clinical trial. Eur Urol 2000;37:161–71.

[9] Koldewijn EL, Rosier PF, Meuleman EJ, et al. Predictors of success with neuromodulation in lower urinary tract dysfunction: results of trial stimulation in 100 patients. J Urol 1994;152:2071–5.

[10] Weil EH, Ruiz Cerda JL, van den Bogaard AE, et al. Novel test lead designs for sacral nerve stimulation: improved passive fixation in an animal model. J Urol 2000;164:551–5.

[11] Carey M, Fynes M, Murray C, et al. Sacral nerve root stimulation for lower urinary tract dysfunction: overcoming the problem of lead migration. BJU Int 2001;87:15–8.

[12] Schultz-Lampel D, Jiang C, Lindstrom S, et al. Neurophysiologische Effekte unilateraler und bilateraler sakraler Neuromodulation. Aktuel Urol 1998;29: 354–60.

[13] Hohenfellner M, Schultz Lampel D, Dahms S, et al. Bilateral chronic sacral neuromodulation for treatment of lower urinary tract dysfunction. J Urol 1998;160(3 Pt 1):821–4.

[14] Schultz-Lampel D, Jiang C, Lindstrom S, et al. Experimental results on mechanisms of action of electrical neuromodulation in chronic urinary retention. World J Urol 1998;16:301–4.

[15] Sauerwein D, Kutzenberger B, Domurath B. Bilateraler sakraler Zugang nach Laminektomie zur permanenten Neuromodulation durch veranderte Operationstechnik und modifizierte Elektroden. Urologe 1998;36:57.

[16] Diokno A, Davis R, Lapides J. The effect of pelvic nerve stimulation on detrusor contraction. Invest Urol 1973;11:178–81.

[17] Griffiths J. Observations on the urinary bladder and urethra. J Anat Physiol 1984;29:61–83.

[18] Ingersoll EH, Jones LL, Hegre ES. Effect on urinary bladder of unilateral stimulation of pelvic nerves in the dog. Am J Physiol 1957;189:167–72.

[19] Scheepens WA, deBie RA, Weil EHJ, et al. Unilateral versus bilateral sacral neuromodulation in patients with chronic lower urinary tract dysfunction. J Urol 2002;168:2046–50.

[20] De Groat W. Anatomy and physiology of the lower urinary tract. Urol Clin North Am 1993;20: 383–401.

[21] Hohenfellner M, Dahms SE, Matzel K, et al. Sacral neuromodulation for treatment of lower urinary tract dysfunction. BJU Int 2000;85:10–9.

[22] Everaert K, Derie A, Van Laere M, et al. Bilateral S3 nerve evaluation, a minimally invasive alternative treatment for postoperative stress incontinence after implantion of an anterior root stimulator with posterior rhizotomy: a preliminary observation. Spinal Cord 2000;38:262–4.

ELSEVIER
SAUNDERS

Urol Clin N Am 32 (2005) 59–63

UROLOGIC
CLINICS
of North America

Expanding Indications for Neuromodulation

Andrew J. Bernstein, MD, Kenneth M. Peters, MD*

*Department of Urology, William Beaumont Hospital, 3535 West 13 Mile Road, Suite 438,
Royal Oak, MI 48073, USA*

Neuromodulation to treat voiding dysfunction has been studied for decades. In 1997, sacral nerve modulation (InterStim, Medtronic, Minneapolis, MN) was approved by the Food and Drug Administration for urinary urge incontinence, urinary urgency-frequency, and nonobstructive urinary retention. The mechanism of action remains unknown, yet neuromodulation has been effective in treating patients who were otherwise considered candidates for radical surgery or deemed simply incurable. Since its inception, widespread use for approved conditions has led to incidental improvements in other areas. Research is ongoing to channel the potential of neuromodulation into other applications.

The major frontiers for sacral neuromodulation in adults are interstitial cystitis and chronic pain syndromes (ie, pelvic pain, prostadynia, epididymo-orchalgia, and vulvodynia); neurogenic bladder from spinal cord injury; fecal incontinence and constipation; and erectile dysfunction. Projects are ongoing to evaluate the efficacy of neuromodulation in children with voiding dysfunction. Other areas that have shown promise, albeit outside the realm of urologic practice, are migraine headaches and chronic angina pectoris.

Interstitial cystitis

Interstitial cystitis is a painful and frequently debilitating condition of the urinary bladder. There are an estimated 700,000 cases of interstitial cystitis in the United States. Its symptoms include pelvic pain, dyspareunia, urinary urgency and frequency, nocturia, and small voided volumes with small bladder capacity. Although some of these characteristics individually are indications for neuromodulation, currently neuromodulation is not approved for the pain component of interstitial cystitis. Pharmacologic therapy for interstitial cystitis includes pentosan polysulfate, antihistamines, antidepressants, intravesical instillations, and narcotic pain medications. Cystoscopy with bladder hydrodistention can provide temporary treatment in a subset of patients. Radical surgery (cystectomy, augmentation cystoplasty) is rarely indicated and may not provide symptomatic relief because of centralization of pain [1].

In 2003, Comiter [2] performed a prospective study that evaluated sacral neuromodulation for the treatment of refractory interstitial cystitis. At a mean of 14 months follow-up, urinary frequency decreased from 17.1 to 8.7 voids per day, mean voided volume increased from 111 to 264 mL, and pain decreased from 5.8 out of 10 to 1.6 out of 10. Ninety-four percent of subjects implanted demonstrated a sustained improvement in symptoms.

Peters and Konstandt [3] have shown that sacral neuromodulation decreases narcotic requirements in refractory interstitial cystitis. Twenty-one subjects with the symptom complex of urinary urgency, frequency, and pelvic pain had cystoscopically confirmed interstitial cystitis. The mean age was 45.5 years and the subjects had failed on average six previous IC therapies. Eighteen subjects were on chronic narcotics before implantation with InterStim and three were on nonnarcotic analgesics. Narcotic requirements before and after the implantation were standardized to intramuscular morphine dose equivalents. Subjects were asked to rate their pelvic pain after implantation on a seven-point scale ranging from "markedly

* Corresponding author.

E-mail address: kmpeters@beaumont.edu
(K.M. Peters).

worse" to "markedly improved" with "no change" centered on the scale. With a mean follow-up of 15.4 months from implantation of the permanent generator, 20 (95%) of 21 patients reported moderate or marked improvement in pain after InterStim; the remaining subject reported no change in her pelvic pain. Mean narcotic use decreased from 81.6 to 52 mg/d (35%; P = .015). Four of 18 subjects stopped narcotics altogether. Patients were overwhelmingly satisfied with the results of their trial of neuromodulation compared with their prior therapies.

In addition to the clinical evidence supporting the use of sacral neuromodulation for the treatment of interstitial cystitis, Chai et al [4] reported that urinary levels of antiproliferative factor and epidermal growth factors that have been shown to be elevated in interstitial cystitis normalized in subjects with interstitial cystitis after a trial of sacral neuromodulation.

Chronic genitourinary pain

Chronic pain conditions pose a very difficult clinical challenge. Multidisciplinary approaches are often used with highly variable results. Chronic pain leads to psychologic disturbances and ultimately to a pain cycle, which becomes nearly impossible to break. Sacral neuromodulation has been used to control a variety of forms of genitourinary pain.

Siegel et al [5] performed a feasibility study in patients with intractable pelvic or genitourinary pain. Patients were excluded if they had definable neurologic or pelvic pathology. Neuromodulation decreased the severity and duration of the pain with improvement in quality of life. Similarly, Everaert et al [6] treated patients with refractory pelvic pain with sacral neuromodulation. They found that 60% of those tested were candidates for a permanent implant and with a mean of 36-month follow-up, all patients maintained a greater than 50% improvement in their pain levels.

Chronic, nonbacterial prostatitis is the most common urologic diagnosis in men less than 40 years old. Typical symptoms include persistent urinary urgency, frequency, dysuria, poor urinary flow, and perineal pain in the face of negative bacterial cultures from the urine or expressed prostatic secretions. Treatment of this condition is often refractory to multimodal therapy. In addition, epididymo-orchalgia is a similar condition where pain in the testicle is prominent without positive findings on physical examination,

urinalysis, or scrotal imaging. Feler et al [7] reported a 44-year-old man with a 6-year history of chronic epididymitis and prostatitis. Pain medications, antibiotics, and antidepressants were unsuccessful in improving his condition. Sacral nerve stimulation provided a 75% improvement in his painful condition.

Vulvodynia consists of chronic vulvar discomfort, including burning, itching, and dyspareunia. Physical examination and vulvar biopsies fail to explain the clinical scenario. Again, Feler et al [7] reported a 71-year-old woman with a 9-year history of vulvodynia, unimproved by medications, biofeedback, and laparoscopic interventions. Sacral root stimulation provided excellent pain relief.

Sacral neuromodulation has been used in each of these chronic pain conditions. Early case reports and small series have shown dramatic reduction in visual analog pain scores and a significant reduction in narcotic use.

Neurogenic bladder caused by spinal cord injury

Spinal cord injury is a leading cause of neurogenic voiding dysfunction. Symptoms are variable, but commonly seen are urinary tract infections, urolithiasis, reflux, obstruction, and incontinence. The goals of management for neurogenic bladder are to increase bladder capacity, control the bladder storage pressure, protect the upper urinary tract, and prevent incontinence. After spinal shock resolves, detrusor hyperreflexia generally develops.

Andrews and Reynard [8] reported a case of a 64-year-old man with T8 paraplegia from spinal artery thrombosis. His motor and sensory dysfunction ultimately resolved, but he was left with urinary urgency and urge incontinence. Self-catheterization and anticholinergic therapy were unsuccessful in improving the symptoms. Urodynamics revealed detrusor hyperreflexia. Percutaneous tibial nerve stimulation, a minimally invasive form of neuromodulation, was performed after baseline bladder capacity was measured at 165 mL. Cystometric capacity after stimulation increased to 310 mL. Serial measurements were performed 3 weeks later and cystometric capacity had returned to baseline. Stimulation was again performed and cystometric capacity quickly increased to 300 mL.

Vastenholt et al [9] reported a series of 37 patients (average age: 43) with spinal cord injury who underwent implantation of sacral anterior root stimulators. At 7 years follow-up, 87% of the study group continued to use their stimulator for control of micturition and 60% used the stimulator for its benefits with respect to defecation. Of the 32 male patients, 65% were incidentally able to achieve a stimulator-induced erection. Overall improvement in incontinence was 73%. Urinary tract infections decreased by 87% after implantation. Forty-one percent never developed an infection after their stimulator was implanted.

Fecal incontinence and constipation

Bowel function is another area of research in the field of neuromodulation. Both fecal incontinence and chronic constipation are difficult clinical entities. Fecal incontinence disables a patient's personal and professional life and can lead to severe psychologic disorders. It is reported to affect 1% to 7% of the general population greater than 65 years of age. Current therapy consists of pharmacologic modalities, biofeedback, and surgery.

Ripetti et al [10] treated patients with sacral neuromodulation from 1998 to 2000. Presuming an anatomically intact anal sphincter, neuromodulation has been shown to improve incontinence and obstructive defecation symptoms. Ganio et al [11] showed sacral neuromodulation to decrease the number of unsuccessful defecation attempts and a reduction in the difficulty of defecation. Further studies have shown that an increase in resting rectal pressure, voluntary contraction pressure, and maximum squeeze pressure can be obtained with neuromodulation. Also demonstrated was a reduction in pressure needed for rectal sensation, first pressure of urge to defecate, and a lowered rectal volume of urgency. Shafik et al [12] reported 78% improvement in fecal incontinence as measured by questionnaire and physiologic-rectometric analyses.

In addition, Chang et al [13] treated a 25-year-old female patient who complained of intractable constipation for 10 years. Colon transit time study and defecography showed nonspecific findings. Anorectal manometric findings revealed impaired rectal sensation. Rectal sensory threshold volumes for desire and urge to defecate and maximal tolerated volume were greatly increased. She was treated by electric stimulation therapy for the purpose of improving impaired rectal sensory function. After 14 sessions of electric stimulation therapy, her constipation symptoms improved

dramatically. Furthermore, the desire and urge threshold volumes were remarkably decreased.

Erectile dysfunction

Electrical stimulation of the cavernous nerve results in increased arterial flow, relaxation of cavernous muscles, and venous outflow restriction, producing erection. Cavernous nerve stimulation has been demonstrated to produce penile erection in monkeys [14], dogs [15], and rats [16].

In 16 men undergoing retropubic radical prostatectomy, Lue et al [17] applied electrical stimulation to the prostatic apex bilaterally, producing visible erection in the retropubic radical prostatectomy population. The authors concluded that it is indeed feasible to produce penile erection through intraoperative electrical stimulation of the cavernous nerves.

Shafik [18] implanted a cavernous nerve stimulation device in a series of 15 men for the treatment of erectile dysfunction. Cavernous nerve stimulation at a frequency of 10 Hz led to penile tumescence and an increase in intracavernous pressure but poor rigidity. When the stimulation frequency was increased to 60 Hz, penile tumescence and rigidity and intracavernous pressure increased, and full erection was achieved. Additionally, Shafik's study demonstrates that unilateral cavernous nerve stimulation is sufficient to induce erection.

Children

Similar to adults, children are faced with various degrees of lower urinary tract dysfunction. Incontinence, overactive bladder, and urinary retention are the most common conditions. Nonneurogenic, neurogenic bladder (Hinman syndrome) causes severe voiding dysfunction and often upper-tract deterioration. The underlying cause is unknown. Children often require management with intermittent catheterization and anticholinergics. Unfortunately, this treatment modality is not uniformly successful and major reconstructive surgeries can be required to manage symptoms. It makes sense to consider neuromodulation before any irreversible reconstruction is considered.

Hoebeke et al [19] reported their early experience with transcutaneous neuromodulation in children with refractory detrusor hyperactivity. Forty-one children, with an average age of 10, had urodynamically proved detrusor hyperactivity and failed anticholinergics. Surface electrodes were placed at the S3 foramen and daily 2-hour stimulation at 2 Hz was applied. After 1-month of trial stimulation, those responding to therapy continued for a total of 6 months. A positive response was seen in 28 of 41 children. After 6 months of therapy a significant increase in bladder capacity, decrease in voiding frequency, and decrease in incontinence episodes were noted.

De Gennaro et al [20] used percutaneous tibial nerve stimulation as a method of treating lower urinary tract symptoms in children 4 to 17 years old. Thirty-four–gauge needles are inserted two fingerbreadths cephalad to the medial malleolus. Plantar flexion or fanning of the toes confirmed proper needle placement. Twelve sessions were performed. They reported 80% improvement in the pediatric population with overactive bladder, 50% improvement in incontinence symptoms, 62% improvement in cystometric bladder capacity, and 71% improvement in children with urinary retention. No adverse events were noted and fear of needle insertion was tolerable and improved considerably over time.

Humphreys et al [21] recently reported their experience of implantation of a sacral nerve stimulator in 16 children with refractory voiding dysfunction. Children with a mean age of 11 years (range: 6–15) with dysfunctional voiding, nocturnal enuresis, wetting, urinary tract infections, bladder pain, urinary retention, dysuria, urgency, frequency, constipation, or fecal incontinence underwent urodynamics. Patients underwent testing with sacral nerve stimulation in a staged fashion and were implanted with a permanent generator. The subjects were followed for a mean of 13 months. Urinary incontinence resolved or improved in 75% (9 of 12); nocturnal enuresis improved in 83% (10 of 12); urinary retention improved in 73% (8 of 11); bladder pain improved in 56% (5 of 9); and constipation improved in 78% (7 of 9). The number of daily medications decreased by 2.8 medications per patient. The overall patient satisfaction was 64% and parent satisfaction was 66%. Two devices were explanted.

Nonurologic frontiers

Angina pectoris

Studies are underway and small series are published lauding the potential use of neuromodulation in the treatment of chronic, refractory angina pectoris. Cardiac syndrome X is defined as typical anginal chest pain with normal coronary anatomy. In a study by Jessurun et al [22] transcutaneous electrical nerve stimulation was performed on eight patients with heterogeneous myocardial perfusion and no esophageal abnormalities. Myocardial perfusion and anginal symptoms were evaluated. Following neuromodulation therapy, there was a significant reduction in episodes of angina and nitroglycerin intake. Perfusion was increased and coronary vascular resistance was decreased.

Chronic migraine

Matharu et al [23] has performed implantation of suboccipital neurostimulators in patients with the diagnosis of chronic migraine headaches. The electrodes were placed superficial to the cervical muscular fascia at the level of the first cervical spine. Neurostimulators were implanted in eight patients with intractable headache pain. Four patients reported complete headache suppression, with rare breakthroughs. Two patients reported very good results, with continued occasional breakthrough headaches. Two final patients reported 50% to 75% reduction in severity, although the frequency of headaches continued. All patients reported a significant reduction in the need for headache medications. Follow-up has been from 7 months to 3 years, and the results have been maintained.

Summary

Neuromodulation in one form or another has been studied for decades for various disease states. Although its mechanism of action remains unexplained, numerous clinical success stories suggest it is a therapy with efficacy and durability. Controlled studies have led to the approval of sacral neuromodulation for urinary urgency and frequency, urinary retention, and urinary urge incontinence. The future holds hopeful possibilities for the application of neuromodulation, namely in the areas of interstitial cystitis, intractable pain syndromes, fecal incontinence and constipation, spinal cord injury, and erectile dysfunction. Neuromodulators have also been used in nonurologic conditions, including chronic headaches and intractable chest pain. In adults and children, in the neurologically intact and neurologically impaired, neuromodulation has been shown to improve the quality of life of those suffering chronic disease states.

Neuromodulation is changing the future of urology. Treatment of voiding dysfunction and likely other disorders, such as pelvic pain, sexual dysfunction, and bowel disorders, will no longer rely only on medications that are "OK" or destructive-reconstructive procedures that suffer from significant complications. Rather, by modulating the nerves, the urologists will treat these disorders in a minimally invasive fashion and neuromodulation will become the first-line therapy before any major surgery is undertaken.

References

[1] Baskin LS, Tanagho EA. Pelvic pain without pelvic organs. J Urol 1992;147:683–6.

[2] Comiter CV. Sacral neuromodulation for the symptomatic treatment of refractory interstitial cystitis: a prospective study. J Urol 2003;169:1369–73.

[3] Peters KM, Konstandt D. Sacral neuromodulation decreases narcotic requirements in refractory interstitial cystitis. BJU Int 2004;93:777–9.

[4] Chai TC, Zhang C, Warren JW, et al. Percutaneous sacral third nerve root neurostimulation improves symptoms and normalizes urinary HB-EGF levels and antiproliferative activity in patients with interstitial cystitis. Urology 2000;55:643–6.

[5] Siegel S, Paszkiewicz E, Kirkpatrick C, et al. Sacral nerve stimulation in patients with chronic intractable pelvic pain. J Urol 2001;166:1742–5.

[6] Everaert K, Kerckhaert W, Caluwaerts H, et al. A prospective randomized trial comparing the 1-stage with the 2-stage implantation of a pulse generator in patients with pelvic floor dysfunction selected for sacral nerve stimulation. Eur Urol 2004;45:649–54.

[7] Feler CA, Whitworth LA, Fernandez J. Sacral neuromodulation for chronic pain conditions. Anesthesiol Clin North America 2003;21:785–95.

[8] Andrews BJ, Reynard JM. Transcutaneous posterior tibial nerve stimulation for treatment of detrusor hyperreflexia in spinal cord injury. J Urol 2003;170: 926.

[9] Vastenholt JM, Snoek GJ, Buschman HP, et al. A 7-year follow-up of sacral anterior root stimulation for bladder control in patients with a spinal cord injury: quality of life and users' experiences. Spinal Cord 2003;41:397–402.

[10] Ripetti V, Caputo D, Ausania F, et al. Sacral nerve neuromodulation improves physical, psychological and social quality of life in patients with fecal incontinence. Tech Coloproctol 2002;6:147–52.

[11] Ganio E, Masin A, Ratto C, et al. Short-term sacral nerve stimulation for functional anorectal and urinary disturbances: results in 40 patients: evaluation of a new option for anorectal functional disorders. Dis Colon Rectum 2001;44:1261–7.

[12] Shafik A, Ahmed I, El-Sibai O, et al. Percutaneous peripheral neuromodulation in the treatment of fecal incontinence. Eur Surg Res 2003;35:103–7.

[13] Chang HS, Myung SJ, Yang SK, et al. Functional constipation with impaired rectal sensation improved by electrical stimulation therapy: report of a case. Dis Colon Rectum 2004;47:933–6.

[14] Lue TF, Schmidt RA, Tanagho EA. Electrostimulation and penile erection. Urol Int 1985;40:60–4.

[15] Lin SN, Wang JM, Ma CP, et al. Hemodynamic study of penile erection in dogs. Eur Urol 1985;11: 401–5.

[16] Quinlan DM, Nelson RJ, Partin AW, et al. The rat as a model for the study of penile erection. J Urol 1989;141:656–61.

[17] Lue TF, Gleason CA, Brock GB, et al. Intraoperative electrostimulation of the cavernous nerve: technique, results and limitations. J Urol 1995;154: 1426–8.

[18] Shafik A. Extrapelvic cavernous nerve stimulation in erectile dysfunction. Andrologia 1996;28:151–6.

[19] Hoebeke P, Van Laecke E, Everaert K, et al. Transcutaneous neuromodulation for the urge syndrome in children: a pilot study. J Urol 2001;166: 2416–9.

[20] De Gennaro M, Capitanucci ML, Mastracci P, et al. Percutaneous tibial nerve neuromodulation is well tolerated in children and effective for treating refractory vesical dysfunction. J Urol 2004;171:1911–3.

[21] Humphreys M, Smith C, Smith J, et al. Sacral neuromodulation in children: preliminary results in 16 patients [abstract]. J Urol 2004;171(4)(suppl):56–57.

[22] Jessurun GA, Hautvast RW, Tio RA, et al. Electrical neuromodulation improves myocardial perfusion and ameliorates refractory angina pectoris in patients with syndrome X: fad or future? Eur J Pain 2003;7:507–12.

[23] Matharu MS, Bartsch T, Ward N, et al. Central neuromodulation in chronic migraine patients with suboccipital stimulators: a PET study. Brain 2004; 127(Pt 1):220–30.

UROLOGIC
CLINICS
of North America

Urol Clin N Am 32 (2005) 65–69

Complications and Troubleshooting of Sacral Neuromodulation Therapy

Adonis Hijaz, MD[a], Sandip Vasavada, MD[b],*

[a]*Female Pelvic Medicine & Reconstructive Surgery, Glickman Urological Institute, Cleveland Clinic Foundation, 9500 Euclid Avenue, A100, Cleveland, OH 44195, USA*
[b]*Section of Voiding Dysfunction and Female Urology, Glickman Urological Institute, Cleveland Clinic Foundation, 9500 Euclid Avenue, A100, Cleveland, OH 44195, USA*

Neuromodulation for bladder dysfunction symptoms has been an important addition to the armamentarium of urologists in the last decade. Pelvic health specialists are interested in the procedure because of the simplicity of the technique and the prevalence of the refractory clinical entities for which it is indicated. With the observed efficacy and interest, researchers and clinicians started developing new technology for neuromodulation through stimulation of selective nerve targets (eg, pudendal nerve, dorsal genital nerve, tibial nerve), but sacral neuromodulation remains the technology most widely used and reported on.

This article presents reported rates of complications from earlier series and shares the complications that have been encountered in the authors' series using the latest technology of sacral neuromodulation: tined lead. The authors have observed that the introduction of the tined lead concept has changed the frequency and profile of complications that were once only technology-related while keeping the patient-related complications of the same frequency. This article reviews the reported adverse events and associated technology, and describes the authors' experience with the latest technology, concentrating on complications and troubleshooting.

Published series

The Sacral Nerve Stimulation Study Group has published several reports on the efficacy and safety of the procedure for individual indications [1–4]. Seigel [4] summarized the reported efficacy and complications in the entire population of patients who had refractory urge incontinence, urgency-frequency, and urinary retention who were included in the trials conducted by the neuromodulation study group. The complications were pooled from the different studies because the protocols, devices, efficacy results, and safety profiles were identical. Of the 581 patients recruited, 219 underwent implantation of the Interstim system (Medtronic, Minneapolis, Minnesota).

The complications were divided into percutaneous test stimulation–related and postimplant–related problems. Of the 914 test stimulation procedures done on the 581 patients, 181 adverse events occurred in 166 of these procedures (18.2% of the 914 procedures). Most complications were related to lead migration (108 events, 11.8% of procedures). Technical problems and pain represented 2.6% and 2.1% of the adverse events. For the 219 patients who underwent implantation of the Interstim system (lead and generator), pain at the neurostimulator site was the most commonly observed adverse effect at 12 months (15.3%) (Table 1). Surgical revisions of the implanted neurostimulator or lead system were performed in 33.3% of cases (73 of 219 patients) to resolve an adverse event. These included relocation of the neurostimulator because of pain at the subcutaneous pocket site and revision of the lead for

* Corresponding author.
E-mail address: vasavas@ccf.org (S. Vasavada).

Table 1
Reported complication with sacral neuromodulation
therapy from the neuromodulation study group

Complication	Probability of occurrence (Siegel series)
Pain at neurostimulator site	15.3%
New pain	9.0%
Suspected lead migration	8.4%
Infection	6.1%
Transient electric shock	5.5%
Pain at lead site	5.4%
Adverse change in bowel function	3.0%
Technical problems	1.7%
Suspected device problems	1.6%
Change in menstrual cycle	1.0%
Adverse change in voiding function	0.6%
Persistent skin irritation	0.5%
Suspected nerve injury	0.5%
Device rejection	0.5%
Others	9.5%

suspected migration. Explant of the system was performed in 10.5% of cases for lack of efficacy. At the time, the generator was implanted in the lower abdomen [1].

Everaert [5] reported specifically on the complications with sacral nerve stimulation. This was a retrospective study on 53 patients who had undergone implantation of the quadripolar electrode (Interstim model 3886 or 3080) and subcutaneous implantable pulse generator (IPG) in the abdominal site (Interstim Itrel 2) between 1994 and 1998. Device-related pain was the most frequent problem and occurred equally in all implantation sites (sacral, flank, or abdominal). This occurred in 18 of the 53 patients (34%) and was more frequent in patients who had dysuria, retention, or perineal pain. Pain responded to physiotherapy in eight patients and no explantation was done for pain reasons. Current related complications occurred in 11%. They performed 15 revisions in 12 patients. Revisions for prosthesis-related pain (n = 3) and for late failures (n = 6) were not successful.

Grunewald and colleagues [6] reported on the clinical results and complications of sacral neuromodulation after 4 years of use. Complications requiring surgical revisions occurred in 11 of the 37 implanted patients (29.7%). They included infections in three cases (8.1%), lead migration in two cases (5.4%), pain at the site of the implanted pulse generator in three cases (8.1%),

and a lead fracture, an electrode insulation defect, and skin erosion at the site of the impulse generator in one case (2.7%), respectively.

Cleveland Clinic Foundation series

Between June 2002 and June 2004, 167 patients underwent sacral neuromodulation at the Cleveland Clinic Foundation for indications of refractory overactive bladder, idiopathic and neurogenic urinary retention, and interstitial cystitis. The authors have performed 180 stage-one operations in this cohort using the tined lead approach. Following 2 to 4 weeks of test stimulation, 130 (72.2%) proceeded to stage-two implantation of the implantable pulse generator.

Stage-one complications can lead to either explant or revision of the tined lead because of response-related, mechanical, or infection-related causes. In the authors' series, 50 tined leads were explanted (27.8%). Most lead explants were performed for unsatisfactory or poor clinical response (46/50; 92%). The rest of the explants were done for infection (4/50; 8%). Explant for response reasons is not considered a true complication as much as it is an integral part of the procedure. Stage-one revisions totaled 22 of the 180 stage-one operations (12.2%). Revisions were done for marginal response (13/22), frayed subcutaneous extension wire (6/22), lead infection (3/22), and improper localization of stimulus (1/22). Eleven (50%) of the revisions proceeded for stage-two generator implant. When the revision was done for a marginal response (13/22), the response was ultimately clinically satisfactory in five of 13 cases (38.5%), which proceeded to generator implant.

Typically, when the patient reports a marginal or equivocal response during the test stimulation in the absence of infection or mechanical problems, the authors revise lead placement with intraoperative sensory testing. The eventual success and progress to stage two of 38.5% of these patients is something to keep in mind for motivated patients with equivocal response. The mechanical problem that was encountered in several patients was a frayed subcutaneous extension wire during the test period. If this complication has occurred after a period of time sufficient for the patient to judge subjectively and objectively the response to the therapy, then the authors typically ask the patient to cut the wire at the level of the skin until either implantation of the generator or explant, depending on response. In rare cases

(6/180; 3.3%) the wire gets cut before adequate time has been allowed, and the authors change the subcutaneous extension wire.

As with stage one, stage-two complications can be divided into explant (generator and lead) or revision. Explant was performed in 16 of 130 cases (12.3%). Explants were done for infection and failure to maintain response in 56.3% and 43.7% of cases, respectively. Revisions were done for infection, mechanical (generator-related), and response causes. The revision rate with stage two was 20% (26/130).

When infection at the generator site is diagnosed, the best management is explantation of the whole system. Stage-two infections were encountered in 14 of 130 (10.7%) stage-two procedures. Most were explanted immediately (9/130). In the remaining five patients, the signs of infection were minimal drainage from the generator site or subcutaneous pain and slight erythema, and the generator was relocated into a deeper or another pocket on the contralateral side in an attempt to salvage the generator. Despite such attempts at salvage, follow-up revealed that the infection persisted in all patients, and eventual explant was inevitable. Mechanical problems encountered with stage two were rare and related to the generator site with rotation of the IPG in one patient, atrophy of the subcutaneous fat in another, and pocket pain in a third patient. All were managed by relocation of the IPG into a deeper pocket.

Response-related complications necessitating revision are more common (18/26) and the algorithm for management of a patient who presents with a decreased or absent response after a successful interval is outlined in a later discussion.

The outlined algorithm includes testing of impedances. Impedance describes the resistance to the flow of electrons through a circuit. Impedance or resistance is an integral part of any functioning circuit, but if there is too much resistance, no current will flow (*open*). If there is too little resistance, an excessive current flow results in diminished battery longevity (*short*). The electrical circuit referred to here begins at the neurostimulator's circuitry, travels through the connectors to the extension wires, through the extension connector to the lead wires, through the lead's electrodes to the patient's tissue, and back through either (1) another electrode and back up the same path to the circuitry (bipolar) or (2) patient's tissue back to the neurostimulator case and into the circuitry (unipolar).

If the circuit is broken, electrons cannot flow. This is called an *open* circuit and impedance measurements are high. Fractured lead or extension wires, loose connections, and other impedances can cause open circuits. Patients generally feel no stimulation if an open circuit is present. When measuring impedances using the programmer, unipolar measurements are most useful for identifying open circuits because they take one lead wire measurement at a time, immediately identifying which connection or wire has the problem.

Short circuits that are reflected in low impedance measurements can be caused by body fluid intrusion into the connectors or crushed wires that are touching each other. The electrons always will follow the path of least resistance. Patients may or may not feel stimulation, which may not be present in the correct area, such as the generator pocket, and which may vary in strength (surging sensation). When measuring impedances using the programmer, bipolar measurements are most useful for identifying shorts between two wires.

Therefore, impedance measurement is used as troubleshooting tool to check the integrity of the system when a patient presents with a sudden or gradual disappearance of stimulation. Many measurements fall between 400 and 1500 Ω. High levels ($>4000\ \Omega$) identify open circuits, and low levels ($<50\ \Omega$) identify short circuit. Medtronic Corp. recommends performing the impedance measurements when closing the incision, at the first programming session to obtain a baseline, and any time a problem is suspected. These measurements will identify which electrodes, if any, are intact and allow the programmer to proceed with programming using only those with acceptable impedance measurements. If all electrode measurements read $>4000\ \Omega$, a revision may be necessary.

Response-related revisions were the most common causes of stage-two revisions in the authors' series (18/26). Among the complications, the authors noted abnormal impedance testing in 15 of 18 patients. A common finding in these patients was equalization of the impedance values in the electrodes where the actual values were within the normal range. A probable cause for such a finding is fluid leakage into the connection. Clinically these patients have reported decreased response, often associated with a spiking or shocking sensation in the IPG site.

The intraoperative algorithm for management of impedance problems includes initial testing of impedances. First, the authors disconnect the tined lead from the extension to the IPG, dry the connection, irrigate with sterile water, and then use the 3F ear, nose throat suction device to dry the connection before reconnecting it again. At this stage the impedances would be repeated. If they normalize, the authors conclude the revision at this stage. If impedances continue to be abnormal one can evaluate or change the 10-cm extension and retest impedances. If they continue to be abnormal, then revise the lead. It has been the authors' experience that the connections to the IPG, or the IPG itself, seldom have anything to do with abnormal impedance values.

Troubleshooting algorithm

After successful completion of stage two, several events can occur, and the treating physician should develop an algorithm to handle these events in a timely and efficient manner. This section covers these events, their probable causes, and the troubleshooting algorithm.

Pocket (implantable pulse generator site) discomfort

The probable causes of discomfort at the IPG site are pocket-related or output-related. Pocket-related causes of discomfort include infection, pocket location (waistline), pocket dimension (too tight, too loose), seroma, and erosion. Output-related causes include sensitivity to unipolar stimulation, if this mode is used, or current leak. To troubleshoot this problem, the evaluating specialist is advised to take the following steps:

1. Turn off the device and ask the patient if the discomfort is still present to differentiate pocket-related from output-related causes. Residual stimulation sensations could last for several minutes.
2. If the discomfort is persistent, the cause is not related to the device output. In the absence of clinical signs of infection, pocket-related causes such as pocket size, seroma, and erosion must be considered.
3. If the discomfort disappears, device output is likely causing discomfort. If the stimulation program used was unipolar, switch to bipolar and see if that eliminates discomfort. Some patients are sensitive to the unipolar mode of stimulation because the positive pole is the neurostimulator itself. Another possibility is leakage of fluid into the connector, which creates a short circuit

whereby the current from the device follows this fluid pathway out to the patient's tissue. Most patients report this as a burning sensation. Although current is following this fluid to the patient's tissue, because some current also may be getting to the electrodes, some patients feel burning in the pocket as well as stimulation in the perineum. Try reprogramming around this by using different electrode combinations. If reprogramming is unsuccessful, ask the patient if the "burning" sensation is tolerable (it will not harm the patient's tissues); if it is not, a revision may be necessary to dry out the connection sites.

Recurrent symptoms

When a patient presents with recurrent symptoms, the authors evaluate the stimulation perception. The possibilities are that the patient perceives the stimulation in the wrong area compared with baseline, has no stimulation, or has intermittent stimulation.

Wrong area

If the stimulation seems to be in the wrong area, the authors recommend going back to each unipolar setting and "mapping" out where the patient feels the stimulation. Set the device to $0-$, case+ and ask the patient where he or feels the sensation. Next set to $1-$, case+ and ask patient again, then $2-$, case+, and finally $3-$, case+. If these combinations do not confirm the target area, start programming bipolar combinations. If those are exhausted, increasing or decreasing the pulse width may help. If one has exhausted the programming possibilities, revision for lead repositioning or relocation to the other side may be necessary.

No stimulation

Check the obvious first. Make sure that the device parameters are set high enough, check for inadvertent on/off (set magnet switch off to avoid inadvertent magnet activations), and check if the IPG is nearing end of life. Next, perform impedance readings, paying close attention to unipolar impedances. Because these impedances measure one lead wire with the case, it is easy to isolate a problem. Using unipolar impedances allows differentiation between which lead wires are intact and which are not. Proceed with programming, using the electrodes with acceptable impedance measurements. Check bipolar measurements to rule out short circuits as well (low impedance measurements). If programming around the malfunctioning lead does not restore the stimulation, the patient often will need revision.

Intermittent stimulation

Check for inadvertent on/off again. Intermittent stimulation can be caused by either a loose connection or positional sensitivity. If you suspect a loose connection, palpating the connection site and re-creating the intermittency is a good clue as to where the problem lies. Taking impedances while the patient reports the stimulation intermittently determines whether the problem is positional (acceptable impedances) or mechanical (when patient feels stimulation go off the impedances are high). Positional sensitivity is when the lead position shifts when a patient moves in a certain direction (eg, the patient reports the stimulation goes away when he or she stands). The lead position may have moved further from the nerve during standing and the amplitude may need to be increased. Intermittent stimulation represents a challenging dilemma to troubleshoot.

Summary

As evident from the authors' series, the complications of sacral neuromodulation have changed with the introduction of the tined lead and the placement of the generator over the back. In the earlier series, most complications were related to pain at the generator site, which was rare in the authors' series. The posterior location of the generator seems to be better tolerated than the anterior location, which could explain the rare need for revisions for pain at the generator site. Lead migration was observed in 8.4% of the original sacral neuromodulation study group series. This was seen rarely in the authors' series in either stage-one or stage-two revisions.

As part of the routine work-up of patients who present with decreased function after a successful period response in stage two, the authors obtain a lateral radiograph of the sacrum; the authors have made the diagnosis of lead migration rarely

(1/130; 0.6%). Spinelli and colleagues [7] reported on the use of the tined lead in 15 patients, and observed no lead migration during either the screening period (average 38.8 days) or during follow-up of IPG implantation cases (average 11 months). The total infection rate in the whole series was 18/180 (10%), which was slightly higher than that reported by the sacral neuromodulation study group (6.1%). Revision rates for stage one and stage two were 12.2% and 20%, respectively. The revision rate in the original study group was 33.3%. Thus, with advancing technology, new problems may arise, but the implanting physician should be aware of the ways to evaluate and manage these complications and appropriately troubleshoot patients with suboptimal responses.

References

[1] Schmidt RA, Jonas U, Oleson KA, et al. Sacral nerve stimulation for treatment of refractory urinary urge incontinence. Sacral Nerve Stimulation Study Group. J Urol 1999;162:352–7.

[2] Hassouna MM, Siegel SW, Nyeholt AA, et al. Sacral neuromodulation in the treatment of urgency-frequency symptoms: a multicenter study on efficacy and safety. J Urol 2000;163:1849–54.

[3] Jonas U, Fowler CJ, Chancellor MB, et al. Efficacy of sacral nerve stimulation for urinary retention: results 18 months after implantation. J Urol 2001;165:15–9.

[4] Siegel SW, Catanzaro F, Dijkema HE, et al. Long-term results of a multicenter study on sacral nerve stimulation for treatment of urinary urge incontinence, urgency-frequency, and retention. Urology 2000;56:87–91.

[5] Everaert K, De Ridder D, Baert L, et al. Patient satisfaction and complications following sacral nerve stimulation for urinary retention, urge incontinence and perineal pain: a multicenter evaluation. Int Urogynecol J Pelvic Floor Dysfunct 2000;11:231–5 [discussion: 236].

[6] Grunewald V, Hofner K, Thon WF, et al. Clinical results and complications of chronic sacral neuromodulation after 4 years of application. J Urol 1997;157. Abstract 1245.

[7] Spinelli M, Giardiello G, Gerber M, et al. New sacral neuromodulation lead for percutaneous implantation using local anesthesia: description and first experience. J Urol 2003;170:1905–7.

UROLOGIC
CLINICS
of North America

Urol Clin N Am 32 (2005) 71–78

Percutaneous Neuromodulation

Matthew R. Cooperberg, MD, MPH, Marshall L. Stoller, MD*

Department of Urology, University of California, 400 Parnassus Avenue, A-633, Box 0738,
San Francisco, CA 94143, USA

Pelvic floor dysfunction is a common problem affecting women and men. This common pathophysiologic mechanism may manifest in diverse clinical scenarios including urinary frequency, urgency, incontinence, or retention; bowel dysfunction; and/or pelvic pain. Existing pharmacologic options for urinary complaints referable to pelvic floor dysfunction remain suboptimal because of the high incidence of side effects, relatively modest benefit, and poor long-term patient compliance. Surgical therapy for what is primarily a functional rather than anatomic disorder does not yield consistently favorable results. In recent years, therefore, therapy of pelvic floor dysfunction by means of modulation of the sacral nervous outflow tract has been the subject of increasingly intense research and clinical applications.

Earlier efforts focused on stimulation of the S2 through S4 nerve roots at their egress from the sacral spinal cord. Although successful for many patients, central sacral neuromodulation has significant drawbacks. Placement of the stimulator is invasive: the system requires trial runs with percutaneous needles placed through the back through the sacral foramina, and ultimately requires a general anesthetic for placement. Moreover, the complication rate is relatively high, and as many as 30% of patients receiving sacral neuromodulators eventually require reoperation. Despite recent improvements, neural leads continue to migrate, limiting the long-term use of the central approach.

Various approaches to minimally invasive neuromodulation have been tested, including perineal muscle stimulation for stress urinary incontinence; perineal nerve stimulation by the dorsal nerve of the penis for detrusor hyperreflexia; percutaneous peripudendal neural stimulation; and direct cutaneous stimulation of perineal, perianal, or perivaginal skin for the treatment of urge incontinence. The profusion of these novel approaches to minimally invasive neuromodulation of the pelvic floor underscores the limitations of the more invasive earlier techniques. The high prevalence of underdiagnosed pelvic floor dysfunction, especially among an aging population, has left a large reservoir of untreated patients, who are best managed with the least invasive successful treatment modality.

The rationale for percutaneous neuromodulation

The posterior tibial nerve is a mixed sensory-motor nerve containing fibers originating from spinal roots L4 through S3, comprising the outflow of the sacral nerves, which modulate the somatic and autonomic nervous supply to the pelvic floor, innervating directly the bladder and urinary sphincter. The authors initially studied potential approaches to peripheral neuromodulation of the sacral cord by measuring skin impedance at various points along the S2 and S3 dermatomes. They identified a consistent area of high impedance above the medial malleolus, which overlies the posterior tibial nerve, and which corresponds to the sanyinjiao, or spleen-6 acupuncture point, traditionally targeted for management of a variety of urinary complaints [1].

Primate studies have shown that repetitive stimulation of the posterior tibial nerve exerts a strong inhibitory effect on nociceptive spinothalamic tract neurons [2]. Unpublished primate data from the University of California, San Francisco,

---

* Corresponding author.

E-mail address: mstoller@urol.ucsf.edu
(M.L. Stoller).

likewise, have demonstrated inhibition and even elimination of uninhibited bladder contractions during stimulation of the posterior tibial nerve. Among cats, S2 stimulation induces excitatory bladder effects at lower amperage, and complete bladder inhibition at higher intensities [3].

The exact mechanisms behind neuromodulation, either central or peripheral, remain unclear. One theory suggests an improvement in blood flow to the pelvis; as yet unpublished data suggest, for example, that afferent nerve stimulation can increase penile cavernosal arterial blood flow. Another possibility is a change in the neurochemical environment of neurons along the sacral pathways. Chang [1] has shown, for example, that after a standardized noxious insult to the rat bladder (1% acetic acid), control animals have a large amount of the nociceptive neurotransmitter c-fos detectable in the spinal cord. If the noxious stimulus was preceded by a session of neuromodulation, however, the spinal cord c-fos expression was dramatically decreased.

Peripheral afferent nerve stimulation in vivo abolishes inappropriate detrusor contractions, leaving the micturition reflex intact. Moreover, the therapeutic effect tends to increase with repetitive weekly treatments over 2 to 3 months, at which point treatment intervals can successfully be increased for durable long-term results and minimal inconvenience to patients.

Early experiences

The first report of transcutaneous tibial nerve stimulation for the treatment of a urologic condition was published by McGuire et al [4] in 1983. They applied electrical stimulation by an adhesive electrode, achieving "astonishingly good" results among 22 patients with a range of bladder complaints including detrusor instability, interstitial cystitis, radiation cystitis, and neurogenic bladder. Eight of 11 patients with detrusor instability were judged "dry" with stimulation as assessed by urodynamics and cystography; an additional two (both patients with multiple sclerosis) were "improved." Four of five neurogenic bladder patients were likewise "dry" and one "improved," and four of six cystitis patients experienced some degree of improvement. These early data, although not rigorously collected or reported, were quite promising with respect to the potential use of peripheral neuromodulation for bladder symptoms.

Four years later, the Stoller Afferent Nerve Stimulator (SANS) was introduced, offering a method for percutaneous tibial nerve stimulation (PTNS) by a solid 34-gauge needle. The method is summarized as follows: the patient is positioned in a frog-leg fashion. The needles are placed bilaterally three finger-breadths superior to the medial malleolus and posterior to the tibia. They are advanced to a depth of approximately 4 cm, at roughly a 30-degree angle cephalad, and in a trajectory that exits anterior to the fibula. Patients experience minor discomfort at the initial skin puncture, but little pain with needle advancement. A grounding electrode (an adhesive electrocardiogram pad) is also applied on each side, ipsilaterally near the medial calcaneus (Fig. 1). Electrical stimulation is typically administered from a 9-V battery-powered generator, at amplitude of 0.5 to 10 mA, with a fixed pulse width (200 μs) and frequency (20 Hz). Confirmation of appropriate needle localization is verified by great toe plantar flexion, or digits two through five fanning or plantar flexion in response to increasingly high amplitude stimulation. On the side with the more pronounced response to the test stimulation, the amplitude is then reduced to a level just below the somatic sensory threshold, and is applied continuously for 30 minutes.

No patient has ever complained of pain during the neurostimulation. Sessions are repeated weekly for 10 to 12 weeks; repeated sessions are required to reverse chronic dysfunctional neural pathways. Patients complete voiding and pain diaries before and during therapy; if they experience significant improvement in their symptoms,

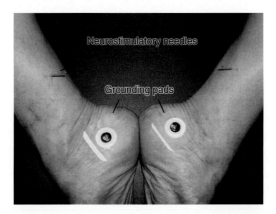

Fig. 1. Frog-legged patient with bilateral placement of posterior tibial neurostimulatory needles in position with ground pads overlying the medial aspect of the calcanei.

the frequency of therapy is tapered gradually after the 10- to 12-week induction period to every 3 or 4 weeks. Some patients have been treated continuously for up to 10 years with treatment every 4 to 6 weeks, enjoying consistent improvement of symptoms. When the SANS sessions were stopped for longer periods of time for selected patients, however, symptoms returned within a period of weeks to months.

In an initial, unpublished experience over several years among 98 patients with urinary frequency, incontinence, and pelvic pain treated with weekly sessions for 12 weeks, average diurnal voiding frequency fell from 19 to 8, nocturia episodes from 5.5 to 2.5, and pain from 6.9 to 1.9 on a scale of zero to 10. Among the 22 patients complaining primarily of urgency and urge incontinence, 80% had at least a 75% reduction in incontinence, and 45% were completely dry [5].

Recent evidence

Trials reported on percutaneous tibial nerve stimulation for bladder neuromodulation as of July 2004 are summarized in Table 1. Govier et al [6] reported the only prospective, multicenter United States experience with the SANS device. Fifty-three patients (90% women, with a mean age of 57) with overactive bladder (OAB) refractory to standard medical treatments were treated with 12 weekly bilateral SANS sessions. Eighty-nine percent of patients completed the study. Seventy-one percent of patients overall met the study goal of a greater than or equal to 25% reduction in diurnal or nocturnal urinary frequency, with mean reductions in diurnal, nocturnal, 24-hour, and excess (>10 episodes per day) frequency of 25%, 21%, 22%, and 70%, respectively (all $P < .05$). On standardized questionnaires administered during the study, participants reported a mean 35% improvement in urge incontinence episodes, a 30% improvement in pain, and a 20% improvement in incontinence-related quality of life (all $P < .05$). Importantly, there were no serious adverse events. One patient each experienced moderate pain at the needle site, moderate right foot pain, and stomach discomfort; all of these symptoms resolved spontaneously.

The European experience to date has been more robust. The first published report was made by Klingler et al [7], who treated 15 OAB patients (11 women) with 12 weekly SANS sessions, reporting follow-up at a mean of 11 months. All patients enjoyed a reduction in pelvic pain (a statistically significant reduction in visual analog scale from a mean of 7.6 to a mean of 3.1). Mean diurnal frequency fell from 16.1 to 4.4 episodes, and nocturnal frequency from 8.3 to 1.4 episodes. Seven patients (47%) were considered to have had complete responses (≤8 voids per day, ≤2 voids per night, subjective cure); three (20%) were improved (8–10 voids per day, >2 voids per night, subjective cure); and five (33%) failed to respond (>10 voids per day, >2 voids per night, subjective unchanged). Statistically significant increases were seen in bladder capacity measurements, although maximum flow rate and maximum detrusor pressure decreased somewhat. In this study, the only to report cost data, SANS treatment for each patient cost €895 (US$770), compared with €10,290 (US$8849) for implantation of the Interstim.

Three centers in The Netherlands collectively enrolled 49 patients (34 female) over a 5-month period, 37 with OAB and 12 with nonobstructive retention (detrusor hypocontractility urodynamically confirmed), treating them with 12 weeks of SANS. Their results were positive and statistically significant, but considerably more modest than reported by Klingler et al [7]. Among the OAB cohort, diurnal frequency was reduced by an average of 2.8 episodes, to 16.5 times per day, and nocturnal frequency was reduced by one, to 2.6 episodes per night. Voided volumes were also increased, and patients reported significant improvements in health-related quality of life (HRQOL) both in terms of general and incontinence-specific quality of life. Among the retention patients, mean voided volumes increased slightly, and numbers of catheterizations decreased, but these findings were not statistically significant [8].

The same group has since expanded to five sites in The Netherlands and one in Italy, and has published three additional papers focusing, respectively, on urge incontinence [9], OAB [10], and nonobstructive retention [11], treating 164 patients in total. Vandoninck et al [10] reported the largest single cohort of PTNS patients to date, accruing 90 consecutive OAB patients (67 female) to 12-weekly stimulation sessions. Twenty-four–hour frequency decreased from a mean of 13 to 10 episodes, leakage episodes decreased from a mean of five to two daily, and mean voided volume increased from 135 to 191 mL (all statistically significant results). HRQOL scores also improved significantly. Among 46 patients undergoing uro-dynamic profiling both before and after PTNS, mean cystometric bladder capacity increased from 243 to 340 mL. The proportion of

Table 1
Summary of trials of percutaneous tibial nerve stimulation for bladder neuromodulation

Author	Year	Diagnosis	N	Criterion	Key results
Payne [5]	1998	Frequency, incontinence, pelvic pain	98	Decrease in frequency, pain	Statistically significant improvement in diurnal and nocturnal frequency, 80% of patients had 75% reduction in incontinence.
Klingler et al [7]	2000	OAB	15	Urgency, voiding diary, urodynamics, pelvic pain	>50% reduction in mean pelvic pain score, decrease in mean diurnal and nocturnal frequency from 16 and 4 episodes to 8 and 1 episodes
Govier et al [6]	2001	Refractory OAB	53	>25% reduction in diurnal/nocturnal voiding frequency	71% of patients met success criterion ($P < .05$)
Van Balken et al [8]	2001	OAB, nonobstructive retention	49	Frequency, nocturia, voided volumes, HRQOL	OAB patients mean 17% reduction in frequency, 38% reduction in nocturia; increased voided volumes; improved HRQOL. Retention patients. Modest, nonsignificant improvements in voided volumes and catheterization episodes
Bower et al [13]	2001	OAB	17 (pedi)	Urge severity, incontinence severity, maximum voided volume	Improved symptoms in 14 or 17, incontinence in 11 of 15, and volumes in 8 of 10
Hoebeke et al [14]	2002	Refractory nonneurogenic sphincter dysfunction	32 (pedi)	Urgency, incontinence, uroflowmetry	Improved urgency in 61%, improved incontinence in 69%, normalized uroflowmetry in 43%
Vadoninck et al [10]	2003	OAB	90	Frequency, incontinence, HRQOL, urodynamics	Decrease in 24-h frequency from 13 to 10, and in incontinence episodes from 5 to 2 daily. Improved bladder capacity, but no overall improvement in detrusor instability

	Year	Condition	N	Outcomes measured	Results
Vandoninck et al [9]	2003	Urge incontinence	35	Incontinence episodes, frequency, nocturia, HRQOL, pad use	Median incontinence episodes per day fell from 5 to 1, 16 patients completely dry. Also significant decreases in nocturia, pad use, improvements in HRQOL.
Vandoninck et al [11]	2003	Nonobstructive urinary retention	39	Daily catheterizations, residual volume, voided volume, HRQOL	Decrease in mean catheterizations from 2.5 to 2, residual volume from 241 to 163 mL. Improvements in HRQOL, especially incontinence-specific QOL.
De Gennaro et al [15]	2004	Mixed refractory conditions	23 (pedi)	Pain, anxiety, voiding diary, uroflowmetry	Improved symptoms in 80% of OAB patients, improved continence in 44%. Improvements in uroflowmetry among nonneurogenic bladder but not neurogenic bladder patients.
Congregado Ruiz et al [20]	2004	Frequency/urgency, urge incontinence	51	HRQOL, voiding diaries	Statistically significant improvements in frequency/urgency, HRQOL and pain.

Abbreviations: HRQOL, health-related quality of life; OAB, overactive bladder.

patients with detrusor instability (70%) did not change, but the volume that triggered instability increased from 133 to 210 mL. Also of note, improvement in urodynamic parameters significantly predicted treatment success in terms of subjective improvement.

Thirty-five patients (25 women) with documented urge incontinence received the same 12 weeks of PTNS, and enjoyed on average more dramatic responses. The median baseline number of incontinence episodes was five per day. After treatment, this median fell to one episode per day, and 16 had no leakage episodes. Nocturia likewise decreased from a median of twice to once per night, and pad use declined from a median of 3.5 daily to none. HRQOL once again improved. Thirty-one percent of patients decreased their 24-hour voiding frequency to less than or equal to eight episodes. There was a trend toward greater likelihood of subjective improvement with increased stimulation intensity in terms of amperage [9].

Finally, these authors accrued 39 patients (27 women) with chronic nonobstructive urinary retention to a trial of 12 weeks of PTNS. These patients decreased their mean number of catheterizations from 2.5 to 2 per day, and their mean catheterized (residual) volume from 241 to 163 mL; their total voided volume increased accordingly. Forty-one percent of patients had a greater than or equal to 50% reduction in catheterized volume. Seven patients reduced their catheterization frequency to once daily; two of these had no residual urine on frequency-volume charts, but no patient became consistently catheter-free. Once again, both overall and incontinence-specific HRQOL improved significantly. Contrary to these authors' experience with their urge incontinence patients, however, in this group increased amperage decreased the likelihood of positive subjective success [11].

None of these studies examined either survey- or urodynamics-based acute effects of PTNS. One paper, however, reported on the acute urodynamic effects of transcutaneous tibial nerve stimulation among 44 patients with OAB. During stimulation, mean first involuntary detrusor contraction occurred at 232 mL filling, versus 163 mL at baseline. Maximum cystometric capacity increased from 221 to 277 mL. Only 50% of these patients had an acute positive response during stimulation in terms of either increased volume at first involuntary detrusor contraction or total cystometric capacity [12].

Pediatric experience

Recent studies have also explored the potential use of peripheral neuromodulation in the pediatric setting. Bower et al [13] treated 17 children with OAB or urge incontinence (mean age 7.5 years, 75% female) in a pilot study of transcutaneous stimulation. Adhesive electrodes were placed for 10-Hz stimulation on the S2 and S3 dermatomes (medial to the posterior superior iliac crest) or for 150-Hz stimulation superior to the pubic symphysis. Children activated the electrodes for 1 hour twice a day. At 1 to 5 months follow-up, urgency had improved in 14 of the 17 patients, and of the 15 with some degree of urge incontinence, seven became dry and four showed some improvement. Of 10 children completing frequency-volume charts, eight had an increase in voided volumes (mean maximum storage increased from 141 to 196 mL). All of these results were statistically significant.

Hoebeke et al [14] tested 18 weekly sessions of PTNS using the SANS device among 32 children (mean age 11.7, 46% female) with nonneuropathic bladder sphincter dysfunction refractory to a variety of prior treatments. Urinary urgency disappeared in 25% of the children, and improved in another 36%. Of 23 children who complained of pretreatment incontinence, 17% became dry and 52% enjoyed improvement in terms of frequency or volume. Urodynamic parameters also improved: 9 of 21 patients with abnormal uroflowmetry curves before treatment normalized after treatment, and mean bladder capacity increased from 185 to 279 mL. De Gennaro et al [15] also used the SANS device among 23 children with a mix of refractory bladder syndromes including OAB, nonneurogenic urinary retention, and neurogenic bladder. They likewise reported improved lower urinary tract complaints in 8 of 10 patients and improvement in incontinence among 3 of 18. They did not find improvements, however, among their neurogenic bladder patients.

Other indications

PTNS has been studied primarily among patients with OAB, urge incontinence, and detrusor hypocontractility. The modality has also been tested, however, for other indications. Van Balken et al [16] treated 33 patients with chronic pelvic pain with 12 weeks of PTNS. Twenty-one percent of these experienced a greater than or equal to 50% improvement in pain as assessed by the visual analog scale; an additional 18%

experienced a 25% to 50% improvement. Total pain intensity and overall HRQOL also improved. Andrews and Reynard [17] reported a single case of a patient with detrusor hyperreflexia caused by a T8 spinal cord injury whose bladder capacity doubled from 150 to 165 mL at baseline to 310 to 320 mL with PTNS. Finally, Shafik et al [18] applied 4 weeks of PTNS treatment using the SANS device to 32 patients (22 women) with fecal incontinence caused by either uninhibited rectal contraction or anal sphincter relaxation, finding improvement in 78%.

Urologists have long recognized pelvic floor dysfunction as a root source of diverse voiding complaints. For patients with concomitant constipation, many urologists refer for treatment of constipation before a definitive evaluation for voiding dysfunction. Conversely, many gastroenterologists advise patients to have their voiding problems corrected before offering a definitive opinion on constipation. Gynecologists faced with a chronic pelvic pain patient with urinary or fecal continence issues might in turn refer such patients for management of these problems before addressing the pain itself. In many cases, these apparently disparate complaints may in fact all be interrelated manifestations of a common functional problem. Many patients with such multiple sequelae of intractable pelvic floor dysfunction may be seen concurrently or sequentially by a succession of clinicians both within a given field and across many specialties. In fact, it may well be the case that all of these complaints may be amenable to therapy by neurostimulation, and that by modulating the underlying dysfunction, the varied symptoms may improve.

Conclusions and future directions

Overall, the results achieved to date with PTNS are comparable with those seen with anticholinergic pharmacologic therapy. Moreover, no major complications of PTNS were reported in any of the studies published to date; indeed, even minor complications, such as persistent puncture site bleeding or pain, seem to be consistently rare. Ecchymoses at puncture sites are virtually unknown. Relative to either central neuromodulation, other surgical modalities, or chronic medical therapy, moreover, PTNS offers a much more economical alternative. Furthermore, some patients failing percutaneous neuromodulation may still potentially benefit from central sacral neuromodulation, and in pursuing a trial of PTNS, no bridges have been burned with respect to eligibility for or potential success of central stimulation.

An implantable device currently under development, dubbed the Urgent-SQ (CystoMedix, Andover, MN), combines the benefits of chronic, at-home therapy (currently offered only by the Interstim sacral stimulator) with the relatively low cost and invasiveness of peripherally targeted neuromodulation. In an upcoming trial, patients with OAB, urge incontinence, or functional bladder retention who demonstrate successful responses to percutaneous neuromodulation will receive the Urgent-SQ implant, which consists of a small (<4 cm), round, implantable receiver incorporating an electrode placed under the perineurium of the posterior tibial nerve, and a radiofrequency generator that can be placed externally on the lower leg. The Urgent-SQ can be implanted with far less morbidity than earlier devices targeting the sacral cord; moreover, implantation in the ankle is less emotionally challenging to patients than targeting the perineum or perirectal areas. This system empowers the patient to self-administer neurostimulation on an as-needed basis, and to increase or decrease the frequency of treatment based on changes in his or her environmental and psychologic stresses. Finally, an implantable device also reduces the required frequency of physician visits.

A number of caveats must be raised with respect to the literature published to date on peripheral neuromodulation. A wide variety of patient populations have been studied, and the inclusion and exclusion criteria used have been variable, as have been both the metrics used to measure responses and the parameters to establish success. Published studies have reported wide variation in degrees of success, even when they used relatively objective measures, such as diary-assessed frequency of incontinence episodes. A need clearly exists for more randomized, sham-controlled trials that use standardized, validated HRQOL questionnaires in addition to diaries and uroflowmetry studies. Although urodynamics offer a measure of objectivity, they may not necessarily correlate with the HRQOL outcomes most relevant to the patient. Sham-controlled trials can certainly be undertaken, treating the control group either with needle placement but no stimulation, or needle placement and stimulation at a location somewhat remote from the intended targeted position. [19] Cross-over designs would also be quite useful. Given the excellent tolerability of PTNS, such trial designs should be ethically acceptable.

Peripheral neuromodulation is a technology still in the relatively early stages of development. How much additional benefit may be realized beyond 12 weekly treatment sessions, the potential use of yet more frequent stimulation, and the ultimate durability of responses are among the questions about PTNS that have not yet been answered definitively. Although most research in the field has been reported in only the past few years, with little long-term data available, the results seen to date are both exciting and encouraging. Fewer patients may respond to peripheral than to sacral neuromodulation, but given the negligible risks and morbidity reported with PTNS, it seems quite reasonable to offer this modality to all eligible patients; those who do not respond remain candidates for central sacral stimulation. A device implantable peripherally will soon offer the possibility of patient-controlled chronic peripheral stimulation, which may produce even greater gains in the treatment of intractable pelvic floor dysfunction.

The ultimate success of neuromodulation will be measured in its success in treating the diverse manifestations of pelvic floor dysfunction, and thereby driving collaborations among clinicians across a range of medical disciplines. The beneficiaries of such collaboration will be the countless patients who so sorely need better therapeutic options to alleviate their symptoms and improve their quality of life.

References

[1] Chang PL. Urodynamic studies in acupuncture for women with frequency, urgency and dysuria. J Urol 1988;140:563.

[2] Chung JM, Lee KH, Hori Y, et al. Factors influencing peripheral nerve stimulation produced inhibition of primate spinothalamtic tract cells. Pain 1984;18:277.

[3] Schultz-Lampel D, Jiang C, Lindstrom S, et al. Experimental results on mechanisms of action of electrical neuromodulation in chronic urinary retention. World J Urol 1998;16:301.

[4] McGuire EJ, Zhang SC, Horwinski ER, et al. Treatment of motor and sensory detrusor instability by electrical stimulation. J Urol 1983;129:78.

[5] Payne CK. Urinary incontinence: nonsurgical management. In: Walsh PC, Retik AB, Vaughan ED, et al, editors. Campbell's urology, vol. 2. Philadelphia: WB Saunders; 2002. p. 1069–91.

[6] Govier FE, Litwiller S, Nitti V, et al. Percutaneous afferent neuromodulation for the refractory overactive bladder: results of a multicenter study. J Urol 2001;165:1193.

[7] Klingler HC, Pycha A, Schmidbauer J, et al. Use of peripheral neuromodulation of the S3 region for treatment of detrusor overactivity: a urodynamic-based study. Urology 2000;56:766.

[8] van Balken MR, Vandoninck V, Gisolf KW, et al. Posterior tibial nerve stimulation as neuromodulative treatment of lower urinary tract dysfunction. J Urol 2001;166:914.

[9] Vandoninck V, van Balken MR, Finazzi Agro E, et al. Posterior tibial nerve stimulation in the treatment of urge incontinence. Neurourol Urodyn 2003;22:17.

[10] Vandoninck V, van Balken MR, Finazzi Agro E, et al. Percutaneous tibial nerve stimulation in the treatment of overactive bladder: urodynamic data. Neurourol Urodyn 2003;22:227.

[11] Vandoninck V, van Balken MR, Finazzi Agro E, et al. Posterior tibial nerve stimulation in the treatment of idiopathic nonobstructive voiding dysfunction. Urology 2003;61:567.

[12] Amarenco G, Ismael SS, Even-Schneider A, et al. Urodynamic effect of acute transcutaneous posterior tibial nerve stimulation in overactive bladder. J Urol 2003;169:2210.

[13] Bower WF, Moore KH, Adams RD. A pilot study of the home application of transcutaneous neuromodulation in children with urgency or urge incontinence. J Urol 2001;166:2420.

[14] Hoebeke P, Renson C, Petillon L, et al. Percutaneous electrical nerve stimulation in children with therapy resistant nonneuropathic bladder sphincter dysfunction: a pilot study. J Urol 2002;168:2605.

[15] De Gennaro M, Capitanucci ML, Mastracci P, et al. Percutaneous tibial nerve neuromodulation is well tolerated in children and effective for treating refractory vesical dysfunction. J Urol 2004;171:1911.

[16] van Balken MR, Vandoninck V, Messelink BJ, et al. Percutaneous tibial nerve stimulation as neuromodulative treatment of chronic pelvic pain. Eur Urol 2003;43:158.

[17] Andrews BJ, Reynard JM. Transcutaneous posterior tibial nerve stimulation for treatment of detrusor hyperreflexia in spinal cord injury. J Urol 2003;170:926.

[18] Shafik A, Ahmed I, El-Sibai O, et al. Percutaneous peripheral neuromodulation in the treatment of fecal incontinence. Eur Surg Res 2003;35:103.

[19] Bower WF, Moore KH, Adams RD, et al. A urodynamic study of surface neuromodulation versus sham in detrusor instability and sensory urgency. J Urol 1998;160(6 Pt 1):2133.

[20] Congregado Ruiz B, Pena Outeirino XM, Campoy Martinez P, et al. Peripheral afferent nerve stimulation for treatment of lower urinary tract irritative symptoms. Eur Urol 2004;45:65.

ELSEVIER
SAUNDERS

Urol Clin N Am 32 (2005) 79–87

UROLOGIC
CLINICS
of North America

Neuromodulation for Constipation and Fecal Incontinence

Michael E.D. Jarrett, MA, MRCS

Boundary House, High Street, Little Milton, OX44 7PU, UK

Fecal incontinence, which affects an estimated 2.2% of the population in the United States [1], can occur passively (without the patient's awareness) or be preceded by urgency. It may result from traumatic damage to the anal sphincter mechanism, idiopathic degeneration of the sphincter muscle, spinal injury, or other neurologic causes.

Constipation affects 3% to 15% of the general population [2,3], with symptoms including a decrease in bowel frequency, abdominal bloating and pain, and difficulty in evacuation. Organic and drug-related causes account for a minority of cases, with most having idiopathic functional constipation. If severe, symptoms can result in impaired quality of life.

The treatment for both fecal incontinence and constipation is primarily conservative. This includes dietary and lifestyle advice (including use of absorbent pads and anal plugs for incontinence); drug therapy (antidiarrheal medication for incontinence, and laxatives, suppositories, and enemas for constipation); and biofeedback (behavioral) therapy [4–7]. Although these measures are effective in most patients, a proportion remains with persistent severe symptoms that require more invasive treatments.

For passive fecal incontinence caused by internal anal sphincter dysfunction injectable biomaterials have been studied. Some benefit has been noted but studies remain small and follow-up short [8].

For external anal sphincter defects, overlapping sphincter repair may be undertaken. Early results show good symptomatic relief in 70% to 80% of patients [9,10], but results have been shown to deteriorate with time, with no patient maintaining full continence and only 50% having improved continence after a median of 5 years [11]. The dynamic graciloplasty procedure and artificial bowel sphincter implants may be attempted to improve continence, but both are major sphincter operations that have a high morbidity and failure rate [12,13]. Permanent stoma placement is another surgical option.

For constipation the surgical options include either partial bowel resection or stoma. Although subtotal colectomy and ileorectal anastomosis is the most widely accepted surgical procedure, it has a significant associated morbidity: one third of patients are left with diarrhea, 10% remain constipated, and 10% eventually progress to permanent ileostomy in the long term [14]. Stoma formation is not an attractive option for most patients and symptoms of abdominal pain and bloating may persist [15].

Sacral neuromodulation (SNM) is a minimally invasive surgical technique that has been developed for the treatment of fecal incontinence over the last 10 years. It seems to be an effective therapy, with reports of low morbidity and sustained benefit, at least in the medium term. Its use in constipation has been reported but numbers remain small and follow-up short.

Sacral neuromodulation

Tanagho and Schmidt [16] implanted the first sacral nerve stimulators in 1981 for the treatment of urinary urge incontinence and nonobstructive

St. Mark's Hospital has received financial support from Medtronic for studies in the past. This article, however, has been conducted without the influence of Medtronic.

E-mail address: michael_jarrett@totalise.co.uk (M.E.D. Jarrett).

urinary retention. A beneficial effect in relation to concurrent bowel symptoms was subsequently noted in some patients treated for urinary disorders [17], and on the basis of this SNM was investigated for the treatment of bowel dysfunction.

SNM has been used to treat patients with fecal incontinence since 1995 and in most series they have been required to have at least one fecal incontinent episode per week to either solid or liquid stool and to have failed maximal conservative therapy. Specific inclusion and exclusion criteria that have been followed by most centers are outlined in Box 1.

The indications have evolved with time and patients with fecal incontinence caused by idiopathic sphincter degeneration [7,18], iatrogenic internal sphincter damage [19], partial spinal cord injury [7], scleroderma [20], post rectal prolapse repair [19], or low anterior resection [21–23] of the rectum have been reported to have benefited from SNM.

The first evidence that SNM might be beneficial for patients with idiopathic constipation was from a series of 250 patients with a permanent SNM implant for bladder dysfunction. Data were collected retrospectively on 36 patients who had concomitant constipation. It was noted that 78% of these experienced an increase in bowel frequency and subjective improvement in defecation (Medtronic, Minneapolis, MN, unpublished data). Other reports concerning the use of SNM for urge urinary incontinence have also included instances of having helped patients with constipation [24].

Evolution of the technique

The technique for implantation of both temporary (peripheral nerve evaluation [PNE]) and permanent SNM devices has been previously described in detail [25]. Modifications have occurred over time, however, and there have been minor variations in approach between centers.

In the past PNE test stimulation used a percutaneous wire electrode (Medtronic model 041830) that attached to a portable stimulator (Medtronic model 3625). This wire was easily dislodged and led to some patients having a permanent electrode (Medtronic model 3080) implanted at open operation for temporary test stimulation, with connection to an external stimulator using an extension cable. The extension cable was removed

---

Box 1. Patient selection criteria

Inclusion criteria
Signed informed consent
Age 18 to 75 years
Greater than or equal to one episode of fecal incontinence per week (assessed by means of a baseline bowel habit diary)
Intact external sphincter with or without previous repair
Failed conservative therapy (antidiarrheals or biofeedback)

Exclusion criteria
Congenital anorectal malformations
Rectal surgery done less than 12 months ago (<24 months for cancer)
Present external rectal prolapse
Chronic bowel diseases (eg, inflammatory bowel disease)
Chronic diarrhea, unmanageable by diet or drugs
Altered bowel habit associated with abdominal pain
Stoma in situ
Neurologic diseases (eg, diabetic neuropathy, multiple sclerosis, or Parkinson's disease)
Bleeding complications
Pregnancy
Anatomic limitations preventing placement of an electrode
Skin disease risking infection (eg, pyoderma, pilonidal sinus)
Psychiatric or physical inability to comply with the study protocol

---

before the subsequent permanent implantable pulse generator (IPG) (Medtronic model 3023) was connected to the fixed electrode, to minimize the risk of infection. Subsequently, a helical wire electrode (Medtronic model 3057) was developed that, because of its increased flexibility and ability to stretch, has led to a reduction in the number of premature dislodgements. The helical test wire is now the most commonly used test method in the United Kingdom [19] and is a relatively inexpensive way of selecting appropriate patients for definitive implantation.

If infection or inflammation occurs the test lead should be removed. The helical wire can be removed without the need for an anesthetic. If the lead is removed prematurely, before a decision can be made about efficacy, a fresh lead can be placed and the patient retested.

Permanent electrodes are now placed using a percutaneous technique [26], necessitating only a small skin incision to place a tined lead (Medtronic model 3093). This lead incorporates plastic tines to prevent electrode displacement. An incision is still required to make a subcutaneous pocket for the IPG.

Lead pain occurred in three patients when the IPGs were placed abdominally. This occurred at the point where the leads were tunneled sub-cutaneously over the iliac crest. Local anesthetic and steroid injections resolved the problem in all cases. Modifying the procedure by implanting the IPG below the superficial fascia in the buttock rather than in the anterior abdominal wall has eliminated the occurrence of this particular com-plication. Placing the IPG away from the midline minimizes the patient feeling the IPG when lying or sitting down. Operative time has been reduced by both the percutaneous technique of permanent electrode placement, and by placing the IPG in the buttock, which eliminates the need to turn the patient during the operation.

With the permanent lead and IPG placement the main potential complication is infection. Once the device has been removed and the infection has settled a further implant can be placed. Judicious use of preoperative and postoperative antibiotics and a strict aseptic technique should serve to minimize the risk of infection. A solution of gentamicin, 80 mg in 500 mL normal saline, can be used to soak all implanted equipment.

The use of bilateral foramen electrodes has been reported in one patient, both for temporary and permanent implants [21]. A dual-channel impulse generator was used for the permanent system. A mild improvement was noted in this patient with bilateral compared with unilateral stimulation, although further work is required to evaluate fully this innovation.

Settings

In studies to date the external stimulator or IPG has been set at a frequency of between 10 and 25 Hz, with a pulse width of 210 μs and amplitude set just below or above the threshold of patient sensation. The sensations felt by the patient include a tingling or tapping in the buttock,

anus, down the leg, or in the vagina in women. There are four electrodes on each permanent wire, each of which can be set as the anode or cathode. Electrode polarity is determined by the setting at which the lowest amplitude is required for the patient to feel the stimulation. The IPG is no longer used as an anode because this led to pain at the implantation site. If the facility to turn the IPG on and off using a magnet is switched off using the patient programmer, potential interfer-ence from environmental electromagnetic forces is reduced.

Review of the literature

Six case series set in Austria [7], France [27], Germany [23], Italy [18], The Netherlands [22], and the United Kingdom [19] and a double-blind crossover study [28] make up the most recent publications on the use of SNM for fecal in-continence. Most commonly there is only a single group publishing from each country and as such only the most recent published report from each country should be taken into account to avoid double-counting patients. The recently published European prospective multicenter (eight institu-tions) trial [29] is not included because a pro-portion of these patients are also included in the single case series data.

For constipation two case series of patients undergoing PNE evaluation only [30,31], two case series of permanently implanted patients [32,33], and a double-blind crossover study [34] are avail-able. The case series were set in the United Kingdom and Italy.

Fecal incontinence

SNM for fecal incontinence is not effective for all patients eligible for the procedure and PNE test stimulation for a 2- to 3-week period allows selection of those patients for whom permanent SNM is likely to be effective. Studies to date include 266 patients, all of who failed maximal conservative therapy, and who had been enrolled and received PNE. One hundred and forty-nine patients (56%) went on to receive permanent implants following successful test stimulation (Table 1). One study only included patients who went on to permanent implantation, hence an apparent rate of progression from PNE to per-manent implantation of 100% [23]. Uludag et al [22], Jarrett et al [19], and Rosen et al [7] had

Table 1
Number of test procedures proceeding to permanent implantation

Study	Months of follow-up (range)	Received PNEs	Received permanent implants (%)
Ganio (2002)	25.6[b] (1–56)	116	31 (27)
Jarrett (2003)	12[a] (1–72)	59	46 (78)
Leroi (2001)	6	11	6 (55)
Matzel (2003)	32.5[a] (3–99)	16	16 (100)
Rosen (2001)	15[a] (3–26)	20	16 (80)
Uludag (2002)	11[b]	44	34 (77)
Total	—	266	149 (56)

Abbreviation: PNE, peripheral nerve evaluation.
[a] Median.
[b] Mean.

similar permanent implantation rates of 77%, 78%, and 80%, respectively, of patients tested by PNE. Leroi et al [27] and Ganio et al [18] had lower permanent implantation rates of 55% and 27%, respectively, although Ganio et al [18] reported five patients with a successful PNE who refused a permanent implant. Studies seem to demonstrate a good correlation between temporary and permanent stimulation outcomes.

Patients with fecal incontinence related to a range of etiologies have been shown to benefit from SNM in these studies. These are reported in Table 2. Studies, however, largely present aggregated data for the case series as a whole making meaningful comparisons between different patient subgroups difficult. A series of five female patients with fecal incontinence secondary to scleroderma are reported. [20]. Four went on to permanent implantation and all were fully continent to solid and liquid stool at a median (range) follow-up of 24 (6–60) months. Apart from this specific group being examined in more detail, published information is lacking on the relative effectiveness of SNM for fecal incontinence in other patient groups.

Complete continence to solid and liquid motion was reported in 41% to 75% of patients, whereas there was an equal to or greater than 50% improvement in the number of incontinent episodes in 75% to 94% of patients after permanent implantation (Table 3). Ability to defer defecation was also improved following SNM insertion and results are shown in Table 4.

The Cleveland Clinic scoring system [35] has also been used to grade fecal incontinence. The score takes account of incontinent episodes (solid, liquid, and flatus); pad use; and lifestyle impairment. Three studies [18,19,23] used this scoring

system and all showed a significant improvement (see Table 4).

Improvement in quality of life has been an important outcome measure in most studies. Fecal incontinence–specific American Society of Colon and Rectal Surgery quality of life evaluation has been documented in three studies with two [7,19] reporting significant improvement in all categories. Two studies reported Short Form-36 Health Survey quality of life questionnaire results. One study [19] showed significant improvement in five out of the eight subgroups (general health, vitality, social function, emotional role, and mental health).

The role of anorectal physiologic measurements in patient selection or outcome evaluation remains unclear. Larger series show a significant increase in squeeze pressure and heightened rectal sensation. An increase in squeeze pressure, however, is not seen in all patients who get a beneficial response from SNM, suggesting that this is not the primary mode of action.

The UK crossover study [28] involved two female patients aged 65 and 61, and was considered to be a randomized study. The patients had received permanent implants 9 months previously. The cause of their fecal incontinence was degeneration of the internal anal sphincter (one related to scleroderma and the other idiopathic). Each patient's stimulator was turned on for 2 weeks and off for 2 weeks, or vice versa. The main investigator and the patients were blinded as to whether the stimulator was turned on or off; the stimulators were set at subthreshold levels so that the patients were unaware as to their status. The two patients were similar at baseline in terms of prognostic factors and both were treated in the same way. Fecal incontinent episodes improved

Table 2
Etiology of fecal incontinence in the case series

Etiology	Ganio	Jarrett	Leroi	Matzel	Rosen	Uludag	Total
Idiopathic	15	7	2	2	5	—	31
Obstetric	—	25	3	2	—	—	30
Surgery	10	8	1	9	—	—	28
Fistula, hemorrhoidectomy and banding, lateral sphincterotomy, rectocele repair, abdominal rectopexy, prolapse surgery, duhamel for hirschprung's, vaginal hysterectomy, post partum sphincteroplasty							
Scleroderma	1	4	—	—	—	—	5
Spinal cord trauma for pathology	4	2	—	2	8	3	19
(multiple sclerosis, whiplash, Friedreich's ataxia)							
Low anterior resection	—	—	—	1	—	2	3
Missing	1	—	—	—	3	29	33
Total	31	46	6	16	16	34	149

from 2 and 10 per week with the stimulator off to 1 and 0 per week with the stimulator on. The study demonstrated maintained reversible benefit at 9 months.

Adverse events

A total of 149 permanent implants were inserted, with 19 adverse events reported. Most important were the three patients (2%) from the same center [7] who developed implant infection within 3 months of their operation. Each patient required implant removal. One patient subsequently underwent reimplantation and the other two patients were considered to be suitable candidates for reimplantation.

Leads became dislodged on eight occasions in seven patients. Five of the eight leads were reimplanted, one of which dislodged for a second

Table 3
Improvement in fecal incontinence following sacral nerve stimulation

Study	% fully continent	% >50% improved
Ganio (2002)	—	—
Jarrett (2003)	41.3 (19/46)	95.7 (44/46)
Leroi (2001)	50 (2/4)	75 (3/4)
Matzel (2003)	75 (12/16)	94 (15/16)
Rosen (2001)	—	100 (16/16)
Uludag (2002)	—	—
Total	48 (32/66)	95 (78/82)

time and was removed. One permanent stimulating device (IPG) was removed because the patient did not wish to have the electrode reimplanted and one was awaiting reassessment at the time of reporting. There was also interruption of the electrode lead in one patient, necessitating replacement.

Six patients complained of pain relating to their implant. Three of these had pain from the lead running subcutaneously over the iliac crest to the IPG placed in the abdominal wall. Injection of local anesthetic and steroid resolved the problem in all cases. One patient had pain over the IPG when it had been set as the anode. Setting the IPG to neutral, using the external telemetry device, resolved the pain. Two patients' pain characteristics and management remained unspecified. One superficial wound dehiscence was reported, which healed uneventfully.

No adverse effect was reported on any patient's urinary or sexual function. The study by Leroi et al [27], however, reported that of three fecally incontinent patients with concomitant urinary stress incontinence no patient showed any improvement in urinary symptoms. Of two patients with fecal incontinence and detrusor overactivity, urinary urgency improved in one.

In the included studies, no adverse event led to any longstanding problems for patients. All of the complications that arose were rectified. Because the fully implanted system is made up of three constituent parts (electrode, short extension lead,

Table 4
Fecal incontinence outcome measures following sacral nerve stimulation

Study	Fecal incontinent episodes per week		Cleveland Incontinence Score		Ability to defer defecation (min)	
	Baseline	Follow-up	Baseline	Follow-up	Baseline	Follow-up
Ganio (2002)	7.5[b] (1–11)	0.15[b] (0–2)	14.6[b] (6–20)	4.2[b] (3–9) $P < .01$	—	—
Jarrett (2003)	7.5[a] (1–78)	1[a] (0–39) $P < .0001$	14[a] (5–20) [N = 27]	6[a] (1–12) [N = 27] $P < .0001$	<1[a] (0–5) [N = 39]	5–15[a] (1->15) [N = 39] $P < .0001$
Leroi (2001)	3[b] (+/− 2.7)	0.5[b] (+/− 0.6)	—	—	0.25[b] (+/− 0.5)	19[b] (+/− 13.9)
Matzel (2003)	40% of movements	0% of movements $P = .001$	17 (11–20)	5[a] (0–15) $P = .003$	—	—
Rosen (2001)	2[a] (1–5)	0.67[a] (0–1.67)	—	—	2[a] (0–5)	7.5[a] (2–15)
Uludag (2002)	8.66[a]	0.67[a]	—	—	Mean 10–15 min at latest follow-up. No baseline data given.	
Total	—	—	—	—	—	—

[a] Median.
[b] Mean.

IPG), a single section can be replaced if it becomes dislodged, malfunctions, or the battery life expires in the IPG. The battery life is thought to be about 6 to 8 years depending on the settings.

Constipation

Twenty patients with idiopathic constipation with permanently implanted SNM have been reported in two case series [32,33]. Ganio et al [32] reported on 16 permanently implanted patients (3 male, 13 female) who had demonstrated a greater than 50% decrease in difficulty emptying the rectum and in number of unsuccessful visits to the toilet with a greater than 80% improvement in the Cleveland Clinic constipation score and a return to baseline symptoms on cessation of the temporary stimulation. Beneficial temporary stimulation results were reproduced in all but one of the permanently implanted patients with an improvement at 1 year from a mean (range) of 2.1 (0.5–10) to 11.5 (5–21) evacuations per week and a corresponding improvement in the Cleveland Clinic constipation scores from 14.6 (8–20) to 2.7 (3–16) [$P < .01$].

In the study by Kenefick et al [33] 4 female patients from 10 had permanent electrode placement following successful PNE testing over a 3-week period. A good clinical response was gained in three of the four patients at a median follow-up of 4.5 months. The number of evacuations per week improved from a mean (range) of 1.1 (0.3–1.6) to

5.8 (1.3–9.3). The Cleveland Clinic constipation scores improved from a mean (range) of 21.5 (20–23) to 9.25 (1–18) with an associated improvement in abdominal pain and bloating from 99% (96%–100%) to 32.25% (5%–100%) of the time. The patient with a poor response was involved in a car accident 1 week after implantation of her permanent stimulator, and may have experienced electrode displacement; she returned to baseline levels [33].

Inclusion criteria varied between the two studies. Ganio et al [32] reported predominantly on patients with difficulty emptying the rectum and feelings of incomplete evacuation irrespective of bowel frequency, whereas Kenefick et al [33] included patients predominantly with reduced bowel frequency and straining. In this regard the baselines from which the studies began were different. The results of the studies, however, suggest that both evacuation difficulty and decreased frequency of defecation along with their associated abdominal symptoms of abdominal pain and bloating can be improved by SNM. The number of patients and length of follow-up were limited.

The small numbers make a meaningful analysis of anorectal manometry difficult. The trends in both squeeze pressure and rectal sensation to balloon distention with air, however, seem similar to the physiologic changes seen in series of patients with SNM for fecal incontinence.

In the study by Kenefick et al [33], Short Form-36 quality of life was improved in all eight subscales. Quality of life was not addressed in the study by Ganio et al [32].

A double-blind crossover study [34] was performed on two 36-year-old women with slow-transit constipation who had experienced a year of successful SNM and was set at stimulation levels that they could not feel. With the stimulator off and on, the number of evacuations per week improved from one to five and from two to four for the two patients. Abdominal pain and bloating improved with increased frequency of defecation.

These results suggest that the clinical effect of SNM in idiopathic constipation is not related to a placebo effect and the fast onset and offset of the effect again suggests a rapidly reversible mechanism of action as opposed to stimulation achieving its effect through chronic changes in the pelvic floor musculature [34].

Adverse events

Four adverse events were reported from the permanently implanted patients. One implant became infected, requiring removal of the IPG and reimplantation at a later date. One patient experienced pain at the IPG site when it was set as the anode, and one patient developed recurrent cystitis following implantation. Kenefick et al [33] reported that one patient was involved in a road traffic accident following implantation that resulted in lead displacement.

Mechanism of sacral neuromodulation

Trials to date have sought to elucidate the mechanism of action of SNM but this remains unclear. The third sacral foramen has been found to be the level at which an optimal beneficial response is gained most often, although S2 and S4 have also been used. In addition to affecting the third sacral nerve root, S3 stimulation may influence the pelvic part of the sympathetic chain that lies on the medial side of the foramen. The sacral nerve root itself is a mixed nerve containing voluntary somatic, afferent sensory, and efferent autonomic motor nerves. It is likely that each of these components contributes to the clinical effect of this treatment.

At the time of PNE placement, if under general anesthetic, motor responses are observed. These relate to direct stimulation of large myelinated alpha motor neurons that innervate the external anal sphincter and levator ani muscles directly.

Overall the anal resting pressure does not seem to be significantly changed in patients with permanent SNM implantation but an increase in maximal squeeze pressure has been shown in some studies, suggesting facilitation of striated muscle function [7,18,19,23]. The improvement is not necessarily seen on a patient-by-patient basis, however, and cannot be used as a predictor of outcome.

Duration of voluntary squeeze pressure has also been shown to be extended, albeit in a small series of patients [27], with the conclusion that muscle type might be altered. This explanation, however, is in contrast to the rapid onset of beneficial effects and return to baseline levels on switching stimulation on and off, even after a long treatment period [28].

The large Ia sensory neurons have the lowest threshold to stimulation and hence in the unanaesthetized patient the first observation on increasing the amplitude of stimulation is that the patient begins to feel a tapping or tingling sensation in the buttock, anus, vagina, or down the leg. Increased rectal sensitivity to balloon distention [7,18,19] suggests that SNM affects afferent sensory nerves.

The diminution in urgency found in the reviewed studies suggests that contractile colonic function is also altered. Urgency has been demonstrated to relate to high-amplitude colonic contractions [36]. Twenty-four–hour ambulatory recordings of rectal and anal pressure suggest that SNM diminishes rectal contractions, enhances anal pressure slow wave activity, and decreases the number of spontaneous anal relaxations. It may be that changes in sphincter function, hind gut function, or a combination of these lead to improved continence [37].

The balance of autonomic nerve activity is a key determinant of colorectal motility and internal anal sphincter function [38]. Altering this balance may be part of the mode of action of SNS. Laser Doppler measurements of rectal mucosal blood flow, an indirect measure of extrinsic autonomic nerve activity [39], have shown an increase in rectal mucosal blood flow up to stimulation amplitude of approximately 1 V with SNM. This is likely to reflect net enhanced parasympathetic activity or diminished sympathetic activity to the hindgut. A rapid change in rectal mucosal blood flow when switching the stimulator on and off mirrors the clinical finding that efficacy of SNM also rapidly changes with activation and inactivation of the stimulator [40].

It is not known whether there is a central effect of SNM on the brainstem and cerebral cortex because the spinal stimulus may be transmitted centrally and peripherally. SNM has been reported to benefit some patients with incomplete spinal cord lesions [7], but in patients with complete spinal cord transection low-amplitude SNM is not effective [18].

Summary

The evidence is consistent with permanent SNM substantially improving continence in patients with severe fecal incontinence resistant to medical treatment. This treatment has been used in patients in whom a major surgical intervention would normally have been the next stage in treatment and the option of a minimally invasive treatment, with the added advantage of testing before definitive implantation, has the potential to have a major impact on this patient group.

The results of the early case series examining the use of SNM for constipation are encouraging. Patients who have failed maximal medical treatment for constipation pose considerable clinical difficulties, with current surgical treatments requiring a bowel resection or stoma formation. If SNM proves to be of benefit to a proportion of these patients, this will be of considerable importance in terms of their future treatment options.

Fecal incontinence and idiopathic constipation are both conditions in which conservative treatment is the mainstay of treatment in most cases, but for a small proportion surgical intervention is warranted. The surgical procedures available, however, have a considerable invasive component with often little guarantee of symptom resolution. SNM is becoming more widely used for patients with fecal incontinence as series sizes get larger and follow-up longer. Its potential benefit in constipation has been shown in pilot studies but larger trials are still required.

References

[1] Nelson R, Norton N, Cautley E, et al. Community-based prevalence of anal incontinence. JAMA 1995; 274:559–61.

[2] Drossman DA, Li Z, Andruzzi E, et al. US householder survey of functional gastrointestinal disorders: prevalence, sociodemography, and health impact. Dig Dis Sci 1993;38:1569–80.

[3] Thompson WG, Heaton KW. Functional bowel disorders in apparently healthy people. Gastroenterology 1980;79:283–8.

[4] Cheetham MA, Kenefick NJ, Kamm MA. Non-surgical treatment of faecal incontinence. Hosp Med 2001;62:538–41.

[5] Chiotakakou-Faliahou E, Kamm MA, Roy AJ, et al. Biofeedback provides long-term benefit for patients with intractable slow and normal transit constipation. Gut 1998;42:517–21.

[6] Norton C, Kamm MA. Anal sphincter biofeedback and pelvic floor exercises for faecal incontinence in adults: a systematic review. Aliment Pharmacol Ther 2001;15:1147–54.

[7] Rosen HR, Urbarz C, Holzer B, et al. Sacral nerve stimulation as a treatment for fecal incontinence. Gastroenterology 2001;121:536–41.

[8] Kenefick NJ, Vaizey CJ, Malouf AJ, et al. Injectable silicone biomaterial for faecal incontinence due to internal anal sphincter dysfunction. Gut 2002;51: 225–8.

[9] Barisic G, Krivokapic Z, Markovic V. The role of overlapping sphincteroplasty in traumatic faecal incontinence. Acta Chir Iugosl 2000;47:37–41.

[10] Engel AF, Kamm MA, Sultan AH, et al. Anterior anal sphincter repair in patients with obstetric trauma. Br J Surg 1994;81:1231–4.

[11] Malouf AJ, Norton CS, Engel AF, et al. Long-term results of overlapping anterior anal-sphincter repair for obstetric trauma. Lancet 2000;355:260–5.

[12] Baeten CG, Bailey HR, Bakka A, et al. Safety and efficacy of dynamic graciloplasty for fecal incontinence: report of a prospective, multicenter trial. Dynamic Graciloplasty Therapy Study Group. Dis Colon Rectum 2000;43:743–51.

[13] Lehur PA, Glemain P, Bruley D, et al. Outcome of patients with an implanted artificial anal sphincter for severe faecal incontinence: a single institution report. Int J Colorectal Dis 1998;13:88–92.

[14] Kamm MA, Hawley PR, Lennard-Jones JE. Outcome of colectomy for severe idiopathic constipation. Gut 1988;29:969–73.

[15] van der Sijp JR, Raising L, Kamm MA, et al. Surgical management of severe idiopathic constipation. Neth J Surg 1991;43:29–35.

[16] Tanagho E, Schmidt R. Bladder pacemaker; scientific basis and clinical future. J Urol 1982;20: 614–9.

[17] Pettit PD, Thompson JR, Chen AH. Sacral neuromodulation: new applications in the treatment of female pelvic floor dysfunction. Curr Opin Obstet Gynecol 2002;14:521–5.

[18] Ganio E, Realis Luc A, Ratto C, et al. Sacral nerve modulation for fecal incontinence: functional results and assessment of quality of life. Available at: URL: www colorep it 2003. Accessed May 2003.

[19] Jarrett ME, Varma JS, Duthie GS, et al. Sacral nerve stimulation for faecal incontinence in the UK. Br J Surg 2004;91:755–61.

[20] Kenefick NJ, Vaizey CJ, Nicholls RJ, et al. Sacral nerve stimulation for faecal incontinence due to systemic sclerosis. Gut 2002;51:881–3.

[21] Matzel KE, Stadelmaier U, Bittorf B, et al. Bilateral sacral spinal nerve stimulation for fecal incontinence after low anterior rectum resection. Int J Colorectal Dis 2002;17:430–4.

[22] Uludag O, Dejong HC. Sacral neuromodulation for faecal incontinence. Dis Colon Rectum 2002;45: A34–6.

[23] Matzel KE, Bittorf B, Stadelmaier U, et al. Sacral nerve stimulation in the treatment of faecal incontinence. Chirurg 2003;74:26–32.

[24] Caraballo R, Bologna RA, Lukban J, et al. Sacral nerve stimulation as a treatment for urge incontinence and associated pelvic floor disorders at a pelvic floor center: a follow-up study. Urology 2001; 57(Suppl 1):121.

[25] Bosch JL, Groen J. Sacral (S3) segmental nerve stimulation as a treatment for urge incontinence in patients with detrusor instability: results of chronic electrical stimulation using an implantable neural prosthesis. J Urol 1995;154(2 Pt 1):504–7.

[26] Spinelli M, Giardiello G, Arduini A, et al. New percutaneous technique of sacral nerve stimulation has high initial success rate: preliminary results. Eur Urol 2003;43:70–4.

[27] Leroi AM, Michot F, Grise P, et al. Effect of sacral nerve stimulation in patients with fecal and urinary incontinence. Dis Colon Rectum 2001;44:779–89.

[28] Vaizey CJ, Kamm MA, Roy AJ, et al. Double-blind crossover study of sacral nerve stimulation for fecal incontinence. Dis Colon Rectum 2000;43:298–302.

[29] Matzel KE, Kamm MA, Stosser M, et al. Sacral nerve stimulation for faecal incontinence: a multicentre study. Lancet 2004;363:1270–6.

[30] Malouf AJ, Wiesel PH, Nicholls T, et al. Short-term effects of sacral nerve stimulation for idiopathic slow transit constipation. World J Surg 2002;26:166–70.

[31] Ganio E, Masin A, Ratto C, et al. Short-term sacral nerve stimulation for functional anorectal and urinary disturbances: results in 40 patients: evaluation of a new option for anorectal functional disorders. Dis Colon Rectum 2001;44:1261–7.

[32] Ganio E, Masin A, Ratto C, et al. Sacral nerve modulation for chronic outlet constipation. Available at: URL: www colorep it 2003. Accessed May 2003.

[33] Kenefick NJ, Nicholls JR, Cohen RG, et al. Permanent sacral nerve stimulation for the treatment of idiopathic constipation. Br J Surg 2002; 89:882–8.

[34] Kenefick NJ, Vaizey CJ, Cohen CR, et al. Double-blind placebo-controlled crossover study of sacral nerve stimulation for idiopathic constipation. Br J Surg 2002;89:1570–1.

[35] Jorge JM, Wexner SD. Etiology and management of fecal incontinence. Dis Colon Rectum 1993;36: 77–97.

[36] Herbst F, Kamm MA, Morris GP, et al. Gastrointestinal transit and prolonged ambulatory colonic motility in health and faecal incontinence. Gut 1997;41:381–9.

[37] Vaizey CJ, Kamm MA, Turner IC, et al. Effects of short term sacral nerve stimulation on anal and rectal function in patients with anal incontinence. Gut 1999;44:407–12.

[38] Frenckner B, Ihre T. Influence of autonomic nerves on the internal anal sphincter in man. Gut 1976;17: 306–12.

[39] Emmanuel AV, Kamm MA. Laser Doppler measurement of rectal mucosal blood flow. Gut 1999; 45:64–9.

[40] Kenefick NJ, Emmanuel A, Nicholls RJ, et al. Effect of sacral nerve stimulation on autonomic nerve function. Br J Surg 2003;90:1256–60.

ELSEVIER
SAUNDERS

Urol Clin N Am 32 (2005) 89–99

UROLOGIC
CLINICS
of North America

Injectable Neuromodulatory Agents: Botulinum Toxin Therapy

Tara L. Frenkl, MD, MPH[a], Raymond R. Rackley, MD[b],*

[a]*Female Pelvic Medicine and Reconstructive Surgery, Glickman Urologic Institute, Cleveland Clinic Foundation, 9500 Euclid Avenue A100, Cleveland, OH 44195, USA*
[b]*Section of Voiding Dysfunction and Female Urology, Glickman Urological Institute, Cleveland Clinic Foundation, 9500 Euclid Avenue A100, Cleveland, OH 44195, USA*

Botulinum toxin first was isolated as the causative toxin of botulism in 1897 by van Ermengem [1]. *Clostridium botulinum* is a gram-positive, anaerobic bacterium commonly found in soil and can produce one of seven immunologically distinct botulinum toxins (BTXs) depending on the serotype of the organism. These toxins are designated A, B, C1, D, E, F, and G, and are the most potent naturally occurring toxins known [2–5]. Although rare today, human ingestion of sufficient quantities of BTX types A, B, E, or F may cause systemic symptoms of botulism. Botulinum toxins C and D affect birds and other animal species, but not humans [2]. Cases of botulism also have been described by the mode of toxin transmission. These include wound botulism, infant botulism, and botulism from intestinal colonization.

Today, the selective administration of therapeutic doses of botulinum toxin manufactured for medical use has become clinically valuable in many neuromuscular disorders. Urologists have recognized the potential applications of this minimally invasive therapy and have adopted it for the treatment of idiopathic and neurogenic detrusor overactivity, interstitial cystitis, detrusor sphincter dyssynergia (DSD), urinary retention, and prostatic conditions.

Mechanism of action/pharmacology

When isolated from bacterial cultures, BTXs range in complex size from 300 kDa to 900 kDa,

consisting of a 150-kDa exotoxin and other accessory proteins called *nontoxin nonhemagglutinin* and *hemagglutinin* proteins [6]. These accessory proteins protect the exotoxin from degradation. The 150-kDa exotoxin is comprised of a 50-kDa light chain and a 100-kDa heavy chain [7]. The heavy chain of the BTX is believed to be responsible for allowing the toxin to bind to the neuron, whereas the light chain actively cleaves a specific site on a protein complex responsible for docking and release of vesicles containing neurotransmitters from the neuron [8,9]. Once in the cytosol, the different BTXs cleave distinct substrates. For example, BTX-A, the most widely studied form of botulinum toxin for urologic applications, cleaves synaptosomal associated protein of 25kD (SNAP-25) in the soluble N-ethylmaleimide–sensitive factor attachment protein receptor (SNARE) complex of proteins [10]. Table 1 lists the various BTXs and their target proteins [11]. All of the target proteins are part of the SNARE complex, which is involved in the exocytosis of acetylcholine vesicles located in the peripheral motor neurons. The different serotypes of BTX have different protein structures, complex sizes, activation levels, and intercellular targets.

There are four steps involved in the modulation of nerves by BTX: (1) binding of the toxin heavy chain to protein receptor on the neural membrane, (2) internalization of the toxin by way of receptor-mediated endocytosis, (3) separation of the light and heavy chains of the toxin, translocation of the light chain, and cleavage of a specific protein responsible for docking, fusion, and release of vesicles containing neurotransmitters into the

---

* Corresponding author.
E-mail address: rackler@ccf.org (R.R. Rackley).

urologic.theclinics.com

Table 1
Botulinum toxin and target protein

Serotype	Protein target
BTX-A	SNAP-25
BTX-B	VAMP (synaptobrevin)
BTX-C	SNAP-25, syntaxin
BTX-D	VAMP (synaptobrevin)
BTX-E	SNAP-25
BTX-F	VAMP (synaptobrevin)
BTX-G	VAMP (synaptobrevin)

Abbreviation: VAMP, vesicle-associated membrane protein.

Data from Rosetto O, Deloye F, Poulain B, et al. The metalloproteinase activity of tetanus and botulism neurotoxins. J Physiol (Paris) 1995;89:43–50.

neuromuscular junction, and (4) growth of axonal sprouts that form functional synapses and regress as the original endplate re-establishes function [12].

Botulinum toxins exert their paralyzing effects by inhibiting the release of acetylcholine from the motor nerve into the neuromuscular junction [9,12]. Without acetylcholine release, muscles are unable to contract. After an intramuscular injection of botulinum toxin, temporary chemodenervation and muscle relaxation can be achieved. There is also evidence that BTX-A decreases the afferent signals from the muscle spindles, thereby directly reducing the neural activity that results in spasticity [13–16]. The temporary relaxation and chemodenervation of skeletal muscle generally lasts between 3 and 6 months before full muscle strength returns. This effect seems to last much longer when injected into the smooth muscle [17,18]. Clinical effects of BTX injection in the bladder have been observed to last between 6 and 12 months [19,20].

Available commercial toxins

There are three commercially available BTXs worldwide. Botox (Allergan, Irvine, California) and Dysport (Ipsen, Luxembourg) are both type-A toxins. Botulinum toxin type B is marketed as Myobloc (Elan, Dublin, Ireland) in the United States and Neurobloc (Elan) in Europe. Botox (initially marketed as Oculinum) was the first BTX formulation approved by the US Food and Drug Administration (FDA) with indications for strabismus, benign essential blepharospasm, and disorders of cranial nerve VII.

Although there are similarities between the commercial preparations of BTX, there are also distinct differences (Table 2). Recently, the

therapeutic windows of the three clinically available BTXs were compared in an animal model [21]. The therapeutic window is the range of doses that gives the optimal clinical response. Levels above or below that range are associated with a poor clinical response or unacceptable side effects. One factor influencing the therapeutic window of a formulation of BTX is its ability to remain exclusively in the target tissue following injection.

Most adverse events are caused by systemic distribution or diffusion to nearby muscles. Atrophy of a nearby noninjected muscle (quadriceps) was observed in mice with doses of Dysport and Myobloc that caused moderate weakening of the injected gastrocnemius, whereas significant atrophy with Botox was observed only at doses that caused maximal local muscle relaxation. This finding suggests that Dysport and Myobloc show greater diffusion within the lower limb than Botox in this model and predicts that they may be associated with higher incidences of clinical adverse events. These results underscore the differences among BTX preparations and indicate that they are not interchangeable and require clinical experience unique to each product. The FDA states that "units of biological activity of Botox cannot be compared with nor converted into units of any other botulinum toxin or any toxin assessed with any other specific assay method" [22]. Table 2 compares the different commercial preparations and factors that may influence the safety and efficacy of the drug.

Neurogenic and nonneurogenic overactive bladder applications

Although the FDA has not approved applications of BTX in the lower urinary tract, clinical experience with BTX for the treatment of neurogenic and nonneurogenic overactive bladder (OAB) is accumulating. Until such approval is granted, caution must be recommended in the application of this therapy until further definitive studies have been performed.

Schurch and colleagues [19] evaluated the efficacy of BTX-A in a nonrandomized prospective study of spinal cord injury patients who had refractory detrusor hyperreflexia and incontinence who required intermittent self-catheterization. Twenty-one patients were enrolled and received 200 to 300 U of BTX-A. At 6 weeks, 17 of 19 patients were completely continent and could either decrease the dose or completely discontinue

Table 2
A comparison of the different types of commercial preparations and factors that may influence the safety and efficacy of the drug

	BTX-A (Botox)	BTX-A (Dysport)	BTX-B (Myobloc)
Serotype	A	A	B
Complex molecular weight (size)	900 kDa	≈900 kDa	≈700 kDa
Package (units)	100	500	2,500/5,000/10,000
Neurotoxin protein per vial (ng)	≈5	12.5	25/50/100
Formulation	Vacuum-dried	Lyophilized	Solution
pH	≈7	≈7	5.6
Year of first approval	1989	1991	2000

their anticholinerigic medications. The two patients who did not respond were given the lower dose of 200 U. Follow-up urodynamic evaluation demonstrated increased mean reflex volume, bladder capacity, and postvoid residual, and a decrease in maximum voiding pressure. Of the 11 patients who responded to BTX-A who were available for follow-up at 16 and 36 weeks, improvements in urodynamic parameters and symptoms persisted.

A recently published retrospective study describes the European experience with BTX-A in 200 patients who had neurogenic incontinence secondary to detrusor overactivity [20]. Data at 12 weeks demonstrated a significant increase in the mean maximum cystometric bladder capacity, postvoid residual, and compliance. Most patients could either discontinue or reduce their dose of anticholinergic medication. Data at 36 weeks were available in 99 patients and revealed continued improvement in these urodynamic parameters.

Only two peer-reviewed studies address the use of BTX for the treatment of nonneurogenic refractory OAB [23,24]. Rapp and colleagues [23] evaluated the efficacy of BTX-A in 35 patients who had symptoms of frequency, urgency, or urge incontinence that failed a minimum of a 4-week trial of anticholinergic medication. BTX-A, 300 U, was injected in 30 sites distributed throughout the bladder base, lateral walls, and trigone. Changes in symptoms were assessed using the short forms of the Incontinence Impact Questionnaire (IIQ-7) and the Urogenital Distress Inventory (UDI-6). Significant improvements were seen in the mean scores of the IIQ-7 and the UDI-6 at 3 weeks. Symptoms completely resolved in 34%, slightly improved in 26%, and remained the same in 40% of patients. In the patients who responded to treatment, IIQ-7 and UDI-6 scores remained improved at 6 months but to a lesser degree than

at 3 weeks. Dykstra and colleagues [24] performed a pilot study using escalating doses of BTX-B in a similar cohort of patients. They found that 14 of 15 patients reported decreased frequency of urination and subjective improvement. The effects of doses between 10,000 and 15,000 U lasted the longest, approximately 3 months. The clinical effects of the lower doses (2500–5000 U) lasted 19 to 43 days. At the highest dose given (15,000 U), two patients reported general malaise and dry mouth.

At the Cleveland Clinic Foundation, the authors performed a retrospective review of 18 consecutive women who presented with idiopathic OAB symptoms refractory to conservative therapies who underwent Botox injection. The injection technique used is described below. Patients were asked to decrease progressively their anticholinergic treatment within 1 week of treatment with Botox. They were followed routinely at 3-month intervals with a micturition diary, and questionnaires pertaining to quality of life and perception of bladder condition. The mean age was 57 years (range 37–80 years). The results are shown in Table 3 no short- or long-term complications were noted. Primary and secondary outcomes were improved significantly for 3 months following treatment, but the duration of effect seems to be less than 6 months.

Numerous studies of urologic applications of this therapy reveal that BTX can increase functional bladder capacity reliably and decrease urge incontinence in patients with neurogenic bladders. New data are forthcoming regarding the true efficacy of this therapy in nonneurogenic conditions. Until more data are available, controversy surrounding the optimal toxins to use, technique and dosing of administration, and long-term cumulative effects will continue.

Table 3
Patient's self-administered bladder diary and questionnaire outcomes using mean percent change from baseline from a retrospective study of Botox injections for idiopathic overactive bladder

	3 mo from baseline				6 mo from baseline			
	N	Mean	SD	P value[a]	N	Mean	SD	P value[a]
Daily frequency	18	−0.21	0.31	0.011	12	−0.17	0.32	0.09
Daily leaks	15	−0.37	0.46	0.008	8	−0.21	0.79	0.47
Daily urgency	15	−0.36	0.51	0.016	11	0.00	0.92	0.99
Global bladder perception	19	−0.34	0.36	<0.001	12	−0.22	0.47	0.13
IIQ-7	17	−0.32	0.48	0.014	11	−0.12	0.51	0.44
UDI6	18	−0.26	0.48	0.037	11	−0.04	0.61	0.84

[a] t test.

Detrusor sphincter dyssynergia and urinary retention

The most widespread application of BTX for urethral conditions is for detrusor external sphincter dyssynergia. Experience with the use of BTX for treating this condition has led to the application of BTX for other neurogenic and idiopathic conditions of hypercontraction of the urethral sphincter or for cases in which lowering urethral resistance may improve voiding function (eg, bladder hypocontractility) [25–30].

In 1988, Dykstra and colleagues [27] were the first to publish successful results of denervation of the rhabdosphincter using BTX-A injections in 11 patients who had spinal cord injury and DSD. The largest series has been performed by Schurch and colleagues [28]. The authors evaluated three different protocols and two formulations of botulinum toxin in 24 spinal cord injury patients with clinical and urodynamic evidence of DSD. Eighty-seven percent of the patients displayed significant improvement regardless of the protocol or formulation used. The mean maximum urethral pressure during DSD decreased by 48%, the mean duration of DSD decreased by 47%, and the mean basic urethral sphincter pressure decreased by 20%. Complete disappearance of DSD was noted in one third of the patients.

Two studies have reported on the use of botulinum toxin in patients who have voiding dysfunction and urinary retention. Phelan and colleagues [29] performed a prospective evaluation of the injection of 80 to 100 U of Botox into the external urethral sphincter in eight men and 13 women who had voiding dysfunction secondary to neurogenic detrusor sphincter dyssynergia, pelvic floor spasticity, or an acontractile bladder. All patients except one could void spontaneously and all but two could discontinue the use of

catheterization. Kuo [30] evaluated the effect of 50 U of BTX-A injection in 20 patients (16 women, four men) who had voiding dysfunction resulting from detrusor hypocontractility. Fifteen patients had an areflexic bladder and five had dysfunctional voiding. After injection, 11 patients could void by abdominal straining without the use of a catheter and seven patients urinated with less difficulty. Voiding pressure, maximal urethral closing pressure, and postvoid residual decreased in 90% of the patients. These patients showed improvement in symptoms scores and quality of life at 3 months.

One double-blind controlled study evaluated the efficacy of botulinum toxin A versus lidocaine in 13 patients who had DSD secondary to spinal cord disease [31]. One transperineal injection of Botox in the external urethral sphincter was superior to lidocaine injection, as evidenced by decreased postvoid residual and maximal urethral pressure and increased patient satisfaction scores.

In a retrospective study performed at the authors' institution, 16 patients who had DSD, 15 women and one man with average age of 53 years, were injected with 300 U of Botox (100 U Botox were injected in the urethral sphincter three times at 4-week, not 3-month, intervals). The results are shown in Table 4; no short- or long-term complications were noted. These small, single-center pilot studies have provided novel clinical and urodynamic outcomes. Larger randomized controlled trials are needed to determine long-term safety, efficacy, durability of treatment, and optimal injection techniques.

Botulinum toxin and pain-predominant lower urinary tract conditions

The therapeutic benefit of botulinum toxin does not seem to be limited to muscle relaxation.

Table 4
Patient's self-administered bladder diary and questionnaire outcomes using mean percent change from baseline from a retrospective study of Botox injections for detrusor sphincter dyssynergia

	3 mo from baseline				6 mo from baseline			
	N	Mean	SD	P value[a]	N	Mean	SD	P value[a]
Residual volume	16	−0.40	0.35	<0.001	11	−0.38	0.41	0.012
Daily frequency	15	−0.09	0.26	0.20	11	−0.4	0.32	0.71
Daily leaks	6	−0.14	0.58	0.59	3	−0.42	0.80	0.46
Daily urgency	11	−0.31	0.91	0.28	7	−0.65	0.42	0.006
No. complete retention	10	−0.82	1.28	0.07	7	−0.51	0.75	0.12
Global bladder perception	16	−0.31	0.26	<0.001	11	−0.27	0.24	0.004
IIQ-7	12	−0.48	1.84	0.38	8	−0.34	2.10	0.66
UDI6	13	−0.28	0.27	0.003	9	−0.27	0.39	0.07

[a] t test.

BTX may have an analgesic effect in conditions of chronic inflammation and pain, and has been used to treat painful conditions in the body such as migraines, tension headaches, and refractory myofascial cervicothoracic pain [32,33]. Although the exact mechanism by which botulinum toxin can provide isolated pain relief is unknown, several hypotheses regarding the antinociceptive effect of BTX-A have been postulated and supported by animal studies and cell cultures [34,35]. It is likely that in addition to blocking the neurotransmitter acetylcholine in motor neurons, botulinum toxin can inhibit the release of transmitters involved in sensory pathways [36,37].

Botulinum toxins inhibit the KCl-stimulated release of substance P from a primary culture of rat dorsal root ganglion neurons [36]. Although all botulinum neurotoxins tested (A, B, C, and F) inhibited the release of substance P, BXT-A was the most potent. BXT-C and -F had intermediate potency, and B was the least potent. Significant inhibition of the release of substance P was observed after 4 hours of intoxication with BTX-A and increased for 8 hours. Inhibition then stabilized and remained steady for 15 days. Inhibition of substance P release correlated with the cleavage of botulinum toxin substrate, SNAP-25. This study not only provides a cell culture model for future applications but also suggests a mechanism by which botulinum toxin may influence afferent nociceptive pathways.

Cui and colleagues [37] evaluated the antinociceptive effect of BXT-A after the subcutaneous injection of formalin in the rat paw. Injection of formalin in the rat paw produces a well-established two-phase response [38]. The first phase, which occurs within 0 to 5 minutes, is caused by chemical irritation and tissue injury that directly activates peripheral small afferent fibers and promotes the release of proinflammatory mediators [39]. The second phase, which ensues 15 to 60 minutes later, is believed to be initiated by the release of inflammatory mediators that activate primary afferents or result in the sensitization of the central nervous system through the dorsal horn nuclei [40]. Treatment with BXT-A, up to 12 days before injection with formalin, significantly decreased the local pain response during phase 2 but not during phase 1. Phase-1 pain behavior was reduced only when high doses of botulinum toxin were used. These higher doses, however, adversely affected rat behavior and motor function. Further evidence that BXT-A does not block phase 1 was provided by its lack of effect on acute thermal nociceptive response in the rats. The authors also found that BXT-A blocked formalin-induced glutamate release. Peripheral afferents are believed to have glutamate receptors that stimulate nociception. These studies support the theory that botulinum toxin inhibits neuropeptides involved in sensory and nociceptive pathways. Further clarification of these mechanisms is needed.

The clinical literature regarding botulinum toxin and pain-predominant lower urinary tract conditions is scant. Zermann and colleagues [41] evaluated 11 patients who had chronic prostatic pain. Two hundred units of botulinum A toxin (Botox) was injected into external sphincter transurethrally. Over 80% of the participants reported improvement in pain as measured on a 10-point visual analog scale. Average pain rating decreased from 7.2 to 1.6. Urodynamics were performed before and after injection. The authors noted a decrease in functional urethral length and urethral closure pressure, a decrease in postvoid residual, and an increase in peak and average flow rate.

Only one published pilot study has evaluated the effect of botulinum toxin type A in the treatment of chronic pelvic pain associated with spasm of the levator ani muscles. In this prospective cohort study, Jarvis and colleagues [42] assessed 11 women with a minimum 2-year history of chronic pelvic pain and pelvic floor hypertonicity defined as a vaginal resting manometry reading of greater than 40 cm H_2O. Patients completed questionnaires regarding bladder, bowel, and sexual function; pain; and quality of life before and after treatment. Treatment consisted of Botox, 40 U, injected bilaterally into the puborectalis and pubococcygeus muscles under conscious sedation. Significant reductions in pain from dysmenorrhea and dyspareunia were observed. In addition, significant improvements in bladder function and sexual activity habits were seen. Improvements noted were nonmenstrual pain, dyschezia, and quality of life scores, but the results were not statistically significant. The authors conclude that there is evidence that Botox corrected hypertonicity of the pelvic floor and thus pain. At the beginning of the study, however, the average pelvic floor manometry baseline resting measurement was 57 cm H_2O, dropping to 43 cm H_2O by week 12. According to the authors' inclusion definition of hypertonicity (greater than 40 cm H_2O), the average patient did not have a therapeutic effect. An attempt to correlate improvements in symptom scores with decreases in manometry values was not made. It is unclear whether pain relief is associated with muscle relaxation or whether other mechanisms responsible for pain relief are responsible. Further investigation into these issues is warranted before reaching any definitive conclusions.

In a retrospective study of Botox for the treatment of interstitial cystitis (IC) at the authors' institution, 10 consecutive patients who met the National Institute of Diabetes and Digestive and Kidney Diseases' diagnostic criteria for IC in research underwent bladder treatment with one of two Botox protocols. The first five patients were sedated and treated with a bladder injection protocol of Botox, 200 U, into 20 sites within the bladder using the technique described above, except that the trigonal area was not injected. The second group of five patients had intravesical instillation of Botox, 200 U, diluted in 60 mL of saline without the need for sedation. The outcome of treatment was assessed by the retrospective comparison of data routinely collected in the authors' continual care tract for patients treated for IC. The results are shown in Table 5. Neither mode of therapy with Botox in patients who had IC resulted in a statistically significant change in objective or subjective outcome measures. Further studies are needed to clarify the role of BTXs in patients who have pain-predominant lower urinary tract conditions.

Prostate

Based on a prostate animal model by Doggweiler and colleagues [43], BTX-A injection into the rat prostate gland induces selective denervation and subsequent atrophy of the prostate. Generalized atrophy and apoptotic changes were observed in the glandular elements. In 2003, Maria and colleagues [44] reported significant improvement in subjective symptomatic relief in men receiving Botox, 200 U, injected into the prostate in a randomized, placebo-controlled trial. Because a relationship between genitourinary pain and muscular dysfunction (levator ani or urinary sphincter) exists in women and men, BTX injections into the external urethral sphincter or levator ani may have a clinical impact on symptoms. As noted previously, Zermann and

Table 5
Patient's self-administered bladder diary and questionnaire outcomes using mean change from baseline from a retrospective study of Botox injections for interstitial cystitis

	Baseline (mean and SD)	3-mo follow-up (mean and SD)	P value
Frequency	16.6 ± 4.6	15.0 ± 3.0	NS
Nocturia	3.7 ± 1.1	4.5 ± 1.5	NS
ICSI score	16.2 ± 0.9	18.5 ± 0.5	NS
ICPI score	14.7 ± 0.6	15.0 ± 0.6	NS
UD16	11.9 ± 1.6	9.5 ± 3.5	NS
IIQ-7	7.8 ± 4.0	10.0 ± 3.5	NS
Global bladder perception	2.7 ± 0.2	2.5 ± 0.1	NS

Abbreviations: ICPI, interstitial cystitis problem index; ICSI, interstitial cystitis symptom index; NS, not significant.

colleagues [41] injected Botox into the external urethral sphincter and reported improvement in the lower urinary tract symptoms in patients who had chronic prostatic pain.

Injection techniques

Bladder

In the United States, most physicians have adopted a protocol developed at the Cleveland Clinic Foundation that uses a total of 300 U of Botox for the treatment of idiopathic or neurogenic detrusor overactivity. Each vial of Botox contains 100 U of toxin, which is diluted carefully in 1 mL of injectable saline. The content of each vial then is drawn into a 1-mL syringe. This yields three 1-mL syringes, each filled with 100 U of Botox at a concentration of 10 U/0.1 mL. A fourth 1-mL syringe is filled with 0.5 mL of injectable saline that is used to flush any remaining toxin from the needle sheath at the end of the procedure. Each syringe is attached to the end of a 5-F sheath that has a 5-mm, 23-gauge needle tip on its end (Contigen Injection Needle, McGhan Medical Corp., Santa Barbara, California).

The 1-mL syringes impart the control needed to inject the small volumes of this concentrated solution. The 5-mm length of the injectable needle tip allows the physician to control the depth of injection into the detrusor muscle, taking into account that the thickness of the detrusor muscle varies from one patient to the next. The delicate syringe and length of the needle tip allow the precise placement of the toxin into the detrusor muscle with avoidance of extravasation into the bladder serosa.

The procedure is performed routinely in the outpatient setting. With the patient in the lithotomy position, 2% lidocaine solution, 100 mL, is instilled of the bladder and allowed 15 to 20 minutes to take effect. A 23-F rigid cystoscope is used for women. In men, a flexible cystoscope with a longer injection needle (Olympus needle, Melville, New York) may be used. Each injection site will receive 0.1 mL of the BTX solution, requiring 30 total injection sites. Priming the needle sheath requires approximately 0.5 mL of solution. Six injections or 20% of the total volume typically is placed into the trigone where greater nerve density is expected. The theoretical concerns of developing ureteral reflux or distal ureteral paralysis induced by the close proximity or diffusion of Botox have not been noted in the

authors' large clinical experience nor in the literature. The remaining sites are distributed evenly throughout the bladder floor and posterolateral walls (Fig. 1). Patients on anticoagulation or antiplatelet medications are not required routinely to stop these medications because little traumatic bleeding is induced with the 23-gauge needle tip. A fourth syringe filled with approximately 0.5 mL of injectable saline is used after injecting the last syringe of toxin to flush any remaining BTX from the needle sheath into the area of interest.

The authors' experience in over 250 patients injected for OAB conditions has enabled them to refine their recommendations for the off-label use of Botox as follows. For patients who have bladder overactivity and borderline contractility as clinically observed with elevated postvoid residuals of no more than one third of their bladder capacity, or poor contractility noted on urodynamics in the setting of detrusor overactivity, the authors typically begin with 100 U of Botox as a trial dose. Because age is a known predictor for a hypocontractile bladder condition, the authors use a lower starting dose of 100 U in patients greater than 80 years of age in an attempt to avoid the potential development of clinically significant postvoid residuals or transient retention requiring intermittent or transient indwelling catheter management.

Two recent articles have called attention to alternative methods of administration [20,45]. Some physicians are using a different dilution technique or are performing the procedure in the hospital under general or spinal anesthetics. The alternative method of dilution is to dilute 300 U of Botox in 20 to 30 mL of saline. Each injection site receives 0.5 to 1 ml of solution. Depending on the institution and physician, this injection technique has been performed under local anesthesia, but mostly under general or regional anesthesia. Some data suggest that increasing the dilution of BTX increases muscle relaxation, but this has not been shown in the urinary tract [46]. In the authors' opinion, this larger volume of injection requires a longer procedural time and has a greater potential for serosal extravasations. It also may be a source of increased patient discomfort, creating the need for sedation or additional anesthesia.

Urethral

Because the early experience with botulinum toxin in urologic applications was a product of

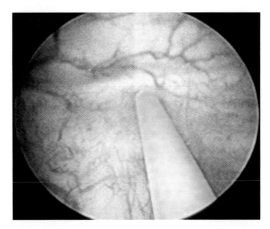

Fig. 1. Cystoscopic needle injection of BTX into the detrusor muscle. (Courtesy of the Cleveland Clinic, Cleveland, OH.)

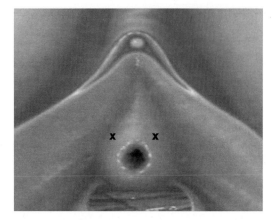

Fig. 2. Placement of 30-gauge needle into the intraurethral wall bilaterally (X) for external sphincteric localization. (Courtesy of the Cleveland Clinic, Cleveland, OH.)

nonurologist interventions in rehabilitative medicine, electromyography (EMG) localization of the external sphincter was performed using neurodiagnostic testing to localize the injection of BTX [47]. In the past, sphincter EMG localization of the external sphincter was relied on in women and men. With experience, however, localization of the external sphincter using rigid cystoscopy, local anesthesia, and patient participation was possible without adjuvant use of EMG needle techniques.

In women, injection of BTX in the external sphincter has evolved into an office procedure performed in the "frog-leg position." A 3.75-cm, 30-gauge needle is placed directly into the sphincter muscle using an intraurethral wall approach. The authors use 100 U of Botox for each patient. Fifty units of Botox are injected into the external sphincter at the 2- and 10-o'clock positions of the urethral wall at a depth of 2.5 to 3.0 cm (Fig. 2). The authors routinely inject the sphincter every 3 months for 3 consecutive sessions and then follow the patient for repeat treatments when indicated by the return of the patient's voiding dysfunction.

Adverse events and contraindications

Botulinum toxins have been used for years as a first line of treatment for various clinical conditions. Local reduction of strength in the injected muscle indicates the expected result. Side effects reported in nonurologic applications generally are limited to local effects and transient. For example, complications after BTX injection for blepharospasm include ptosis, facial muscle

paralysis, dryness of the eyes, and hematoma formation [48]. A flulike syndrome also can occur and has been attributed to the nontoxin portion of the formulations [49].

There have been few reports of adverse events reported with BTX-A injections for urologic conditions. Although BTX-A is believed to remain in the muscle that is injected, rare cases of patients having systemic side effects such as hyposthenia lasting 2 to 4 weeks and generalized muscle weakness have been reported [50–52]. It also may be possible to weaken the detrusor muscle to such an extent that transient intermittent self-catheterization is necessary. Most published studies report no injection-related complications or BTX-A–related side effects.

Most treated patients respond for many years without tachyphylaxis or increases in dosages for successful outcomes. In other chronic disease conditions where BTXs have been used, there have been reports of neutralizing antibody formation [53]. These antibodies may interfere with the efficacy of the BTX therapy, but do not seem to pose any safety risk to the patient. Initial work pertaining to cervical dystonia revealed neutralizing antibody formation in up to 17% of patients who had received multiple injections of Botox [53]. These patients, however, were injected with a previous formulation of Botox that was in clinical use before 1998 (original 79-11 Botox). This original formulation contained 25 ng of total protein/100 U, whereas the currently marketed reformulation contains 5 ng of protein/100 U [54].

Decreasing the protein load and spreading out patient injection cycles by a minimum of 12 weeks have reduced drastically the formation of neutralizing antibodies. In a recent comparison study of patients injected for cervical dystonia, neutralizing antibodies were present in 9.5% of the 42 patients who were injected with the original formulation of Botox. None of the 119 patients treated exclusively with the current formulation of Botox produced neutralizing antibodies [55]. There is only one case report of resistance to BTX-A with regards to bladder injections in a quadriplegic patient who previously had received repeated BTX-A injections in the the bladder and limbs [56]. Resistance was quantified based on the M wave of the extensor digitorum brevis during stimulation of the peroneal nerve. Her bladder spasticity was treated successfully with BTX-B.

Contraindications to BTX injections include myasthenia gravis, Eaton-Lambert syndrome, amyotrophic lateral sclerosis (Lou Gherig Disease), breastfeeding, pregnancy, and the concomitant use of agents that potentially act at the level of neuromuscular transmission such as aminoglycosides. Patients should be informed that some BTX formulations may include stabilizers such as albumin derived from human blood, which may be of religious or cultural importance.

Summary

Botulinum toxin therapy is a diverse treatment option for various dysfunctions of the lower urinary tract. The limited but growing clinical experience reveals that temporary chemodenervation with reduction or loss of neuronal activity at the target organ may be achieved with minimal risk. This highly favorable risk-benefit ratio in urology is derived from the clinical ability to treat an end-organ condition effectively with controllable site-specific delivery (eg, subcutaneous, intramuscular, or instillation) combined with high affinity for toxin uptake by the peripheral cholinergic nerves. Although many questions remain regarding the optimal use of this minimally invasive option for urologic applications, the opportunity for expanding indications will provide urologists with more options for addressing difficult challenges in voiding dysfunction.

References

[1] Van Ermengem E. Ueber einen neuen anaerobean Bacillus and siene Beziehungen zum Botuliams. Ztsch Hyg Infekt 1897;26:1.

[2] Centers for Disease Control and Prevention. Botulism in the United States, 1899–1996: handbook for epidemiologists, clinicians, and laboratory workers. Atlanta (GA): Centers for Disease Control and Prevention; 1998.

[3] Gill MD. Bacterial toxins: a table of lethal amounts. Microbiol Rev 1982;46:86–94.

[4] Foran PG, Mohammed N, Lisk GO, et al. Evaluation of the therapeutic usefulness of botulinum neurotoxin B, C1, E, and F compared with the long lasting type A. J Biol Chem 2003;278(2):1363–71.

[5] Aoki KR, Guyer B. Botulinum toxin type A and other botulinum toxin serotypes: a comparative review of biochemical and pharmacological actions. Eur J Neurol 2001;8(Suppl 5):21–9.

[6] DasGupta BR. Structures of botulinium neurotoxin, its functional domains, and perspectives on the crystalline type A toxin. In: Janovich J, Hallet M, editors. Therapy with botulimium toxin. New York: Marcel Dekker; 1994. p. 15–39.

[7] Brin MF. Botulinum toxin: chemistry, pharmacology, toxicity, and immunology Muscle Nerve 1997; 20:S146–68.

[8] Oguma K, Fujinaga Y, Inoue K. Structure and function of Clostridum botulinium toxins. Microbio Immunol 1995;17:402–7.

[9] Montecucco C, Schiavo G, Tugnoli V, et al. Botulinum neurotoxins: mechanism of action and therapeutic applications. Mol Med Today 1996;2: 418–24.

[10] Rothman JE. Mechanism of intracellular protein transport. Nature 1994;372:55–63.

[11] Rosetto O, Deloye F, Poulain B, et al. The metalloproteinase activity of tetanus and botulism neurotoxins. J Physiol (Paris) 1995;89:43–50.

[12] dePaiva A, Meunier FA, Molgo J, et al. Functional repair of motor endplates after botulinum neurotoxin type A poisoning: biphasic switch of synaptic activity between nerve sprouts and their parent terminals. Proc Natl Acad Sci USA 1999;96:3200–5.

[13] Filippi GM, Errico P, Santarelli R, et al. Botulinum A toxin effects on rat jaw muscle spindles. Acta Otolaryngol 1993;113(3):400–4.

[14] Rosales RL, Arimura K, Takenaga S, et al. Extrafusal and intrafusal muscle effects in experimental botulinum toxin- A injection. Muscle Nerve 1996; 19(4):488–96.

[15] Moreno-Lopez B, et al. Discharge properties of extraocular muscle motoneurons in the alert cat following the peripheral injection of botulinum neurotoxin type A. Mov Disord 1995;10(3):386.

[16] Priori A, Berardelli A, Mercuri B, et al. Physiological effects produced by botulinum toxin treatment of upper limb dystonia changes in reciprocal inhibition between forearm muscles. Brain 1995;118(3): 801–7.

[17] Pasricha PJ, Rai R, Ravich WJ, et al. Botulinum toxin for achalsia: long term outcome and predictors of response. Gastroenterology 1996;110(5):1410–5.

[18] Annese V, Basciani M, Borrelli O, et al. Intrasphinctertic injection of Botulinum toxin is effective in long-term treatment of esophageal achalasia. Muscle Nerve 1998;21(11):1540–2.

[19] Schurch B, et al. Botulinum-A toxin for treating detrusor hyper-reflexia in spinal cord injured patients: a new alternative to anticholinergic drugs? Preliminary results. J Urol 2000;164:692–7.

[20] Reitz A, Stohrer M, Kramer G, et al. European experience of 200 cases treated with botulinum-a toxin injection into the detrusor muscle for urinary incontinence due to neurogenic detrusor overactivity. Eur Urol 2004;45:510–5.

[21] Roger Aoki K. Botulinum neurotoxin serotypes A and B preparations have different safety margins in preclinical models of muscle weakening efficacy and systemic safety. Toxicon 2002;40(7):923–8.

[22] Botox [package insert]. Irvine (CA): Allergan, Inc.

[23] Rapp D, Lucioni A, Katz E, et al. Use of botulinum-A toxin for the trratment of refractory overactive bladder symtpoms: an initial experience. Urology 2004;63(6):1071–5.

[24] Dykstra D, Enriquez A, Valley M. Treatment of overactive bladder with botulinum toxin type B: a pilot study. Int Urogynecol J Pelvic Floor Dysfunct 2003;14:424–6.

[25] Jost W, Naumann M. Botulinum toxin in neuro-urological disorders. Mov Disord 2004;19(S8): S142–5.

[26] Jost W, Merkle W, Muller-Lobeck H. Urethrismus accounting for voiding disorder. Urology 1998;52: 352.

[27] Dykstra DD, Sidi AA, Scott AB, et al. Effects of botulinum-A toxin on detrusor-sphincter dyssynergia in spinal cord injury patients. J Urol 1988; 139(5):919–22.

[28] Schurch B, Hauri D, Rodic B, et al. Botulinum A toxin as a treatment of detrusor-sphincter dyssynergia: a prospective study in 24 spinal cord injury patients. J Urol 1996;155(3):1023–9.

[29] Phelan MW, Franks M, Somogyi GT, et al. Botulinum toxin urethral sphincter injection to restore bladder emptying in men and women with voiding dysfunction. J Urol 2001;165:1107–10.

[30] Kuo HC. Effect of Botulinum A toxin in the treatment of voiding dysfunction due to detrusor underactivity. Urology 2003;61(3):550–4.

[31] de Seze M, Petit H, Gallien P, et al. Botulinum A toxin and detrusor sphincter dyssynergia: a double blind lidocaine-controlled study in 13 patients with spinal cord disease. Eur Urol 2002;42:56–62.

[32] Taqi D, Gunyea I, Bhakta B, et al. Botulinum toxin-type A (Botox®) in the treatment of refractory myofascial cervicothoracic pain: a prospective trial. Pain Med 2002;3(2):173–4.

[33] Smuts JA, Barnard PWA. Botulinum toxin type A in the treatment of headache syndromes: a clinical report of 79 patients. Cephalgia 2000;2:332.

[34] Aoki RK. Evidence for antinociceptive activity of botulinum toxin type A in pain management. Headache 2003;43(Suppl 1):S9–13.

[35] Klein AW. The therapeutic potential of botulinum toxin. Dermatol Surg 2004;30(3):452–5.

[36] Welch M, Purkiss J, Foster K. Sensitivity of embryonic rat dorsal root ganglia neurons to Clostridium botulinum neurotoxins. Toxicon 2000;38:245–58.

[37] Cui M, Khanijou S, Rubino J, et al. Subcutaneous administration of botulinum toxin A reduces formalin-induced pain. Pain 2004;107(1–2):125–33.

[38] Wheeler-Aceto H, Cowan A. Neurogenic and tissue mediated components of formalin-induced edema: evidence for supraspinal regulation. Agents Actions 1991;34:264–9.

[39] Cao YQ, Mantyh PW, Carlson EJ, et al. Primary afferent tachykinins are required to experience moderate to intense pain. Nature 1998;392:390–4.

[40] Coderre TJ, Katz J, Vaccarino AL, et al. Contribution of central neuroplasticity to pathological pain: review of clinical and experimental evidence. Pain 1993;52:259–85.

[41] Zermann D, Ishigooka M, Schubert J, et al. Perisphincteric injection of botulinum toxin type A. A treatment option for patients with chronic pelvic pain? Eur Urol 2000;38(4):393–9.

[42] Jarvis SK, Abbott JA, Lenart MB, et al. Pilot study of botulinum toxin type A in the treatment of chronic pelvic pain associated with spasm of the levator ani muscles Aust N Z J Obstet Gynaecol 2004;44(1):46–50.

[43] Doggweiller R, Zermann D, Ishigooka M, et al. Botox-induced prostatic involution. Prostate 1998; 37:44–50.

[44] Maria G, Brisinda G, Civello IM, et al. Relief by botulinum toxin of voiding dysfunction due to benign prostatic hyperplasia: results of a randomized, placebo-controlled study. Urology 2003;62:259–65.

[45] Smith C, Chancellor M. The emerging role of botulinum toxin in the management of voiding dysfunction. J Urol 2004;171:2128–37.

[46] Kim H, Hwang J, Jeong S, et al. Effect of muscle activity and botulinum toxin dilution volume on muscle paralysis. Dev Med Child Neurol 2003;45:200.

[47] Schurch B, Hodler J, Rodic B. Botulinum A toxin as a treatment of detrusor-sphincter dyssynergia in patients with spinal cord injury: MRI controlled transperineal injections. J Neurol Neurosurg Psychiatry 1997;63(4):474–6.

[48] Janovich J, Brin MF. Botulinium toxin: a historical perspective and potential new indications. Muscle Nerve 1997;20:S129–45.

[49] Muthane UB, Panikar JN. Botulinum toxins: pharmacology and its current therapeutic evidence for use. Neurol India 2003;51:455–60.

[50] Del Popolo G, Li MV, Panariello G, et al. English botulinum toxin-A in the treatment of neurogenic detrusor overactivity. Neurourol Urodyn 2003; 22(5):498–9.

[51] Wyndaele JJ, Van Dromme SA. Muscular weakness as a side effect of botulinum toxin injection for neurogenic detrusor overactivity. Spinal Cord 2002; 40(11):599–600.

[52] Dykstra DD, Sidi AA. Treatment of detrusor-sphincter dyssynergia with botulinum A toxin: a double-blind study. Arch Phys Med Rehabil 1990;71:24–6.

[53] BOTOX® (Botulinum toxin type A, purified neurotoxin complex) product information. Available at: http://www.botox.com/site/consumers/prescribing_info/botox.asp. Accessed October 3, 2004.

[54] A randomized, multicenter, double-blind, placebo-controlled study of intramuscular BOTOX® (botulinum toxin type A) purified neurotoxin complex (original 79–11 BOTOX®) for the treatment of cervical dystonia. Irvine (CA): Allergan, Inc.; 1998.

[55] Jankovic J, Vuong KD, Ahsan J. Comparison of efficacy and immunogenicity of original versus current botulinum toxin in cervical dystonia. Neurology 2003;60(7):1186–8.

[56] Pistolesi D, Selli C, Stampacchia G. Botulinum toxin type B for type A resistant bladder spasticity. J Urol 2004;171:802–3.

ELSEVIER
SAUNDERS

Urol Clin N Am 32 (2005) 101–107

UROLOGIC
CLINICS
of North America

Neuromodulation in Pediatrics

Ahmad H. Bani-Hani, MD[a], David R. Vandersteen, MD[a,b],
Yuri E. Reinberg, MD[a,b],*

[a]Department of Urology, Mayo Graduate School of Medicine, Mayo Clinic,
200 First Street SW, Rochester, MN 55901, USA
[b]Pediatric Surgical Associates, 2545 Chicago Avenue South, Suite 104, Minneapolis, MN 55404-4567, USA

Voiding dysfunction, sometimes referred to as *dysfunctional elimination syndrome* (DES), is encountered commonly in the pediatric population. It represents a constellation of symptoms that affect urinary storage or emptying. Common symptoms include recurrent urinary tract infections, nocturnal or diurnal enuresis, urgency, urge incontinence, posturing, frequency, urinary dribbling, infrequent voiding, weak or intermittent stream, and pelvic pain.

The advent of clean intermittent catheterization, evolution of urodynamic testing, and refinement in surgical techniques for urinary incontinence changed the traditional approach to managing this subset of patients. With this change came a great understanding of the pathophysiology of many disorders that can affect children primarily. A team approach with expertise in different therapeutic modalities, including pharmacologic, behavioral modification, and biofeedback, provides for the highest success rate.

A common challenge, however, lies in children resistant to conventional therapy, causing significant distress to caregivers, patients, and their families. In the last few decades, in an effort to solve this problem, several nonconventional therapeutic modalities have emerged with promising results. They share a common objective of restoring bladder and bowel function to as normal as possible based on the current understanding of the various neural pathways that connect the central with the peripheral micturition reflexes to correct inefficient bladder habits, uncoordinated sphincter activity, and bladder storage problems. This article highlights neuromodulators that have been used in the pediatric population.

Acupuncture

Acupuncture, a traditional Chinese medical modality, has been investigated recently as an alternative, nonconventional method in the treatment of children who have monosymptomatic primary nocturnal enuresis and in children who have hyperreflexic neurogenic bladders. In Chinese literature, success rates of 73% to 100% have been reported [1–3].

Primary nocturnal enuresis is the most common type of urinary incontinence evaluated by the pediatric urologist. It is estimated that 15% of 5-year-old children, 7% to 10% of 7-year-old children, and 5% of 10-year-old children are affected by this condition, resulting in significant psychosocial burden among affected children and their respective parents [4–7]. The rate of spontaneous cure is about 15% per year [5] with 0.5% to 1% of children enuretic into adulthood [5,7]. Conventional treatment options for these children have included behavioral (eg, alarm system), pharmacologic (eg, tricyclic antidepressants, Desmopressin, anticholinergics), or a combination of both therapies. In recently published studies, children refractory to the above measures have been subjects in acupuncture trials as an alternative therapeutic modality with cure rates ranging from 21.8% to 80% [8–12]. Table 1 summarizes these studies. Honjo and colleagues, in a study involving eight patients who had urinary

* Corresponding author.

E-mail address: yreinberg@pediatricsurgical
associates.com (Y.E. Reinberg).

Table 1
Summary of acupuncture trials

Study	Year	Acupuncture type	No. of patients	Follow-up duration	Results
Bjorkstrom and colleagues	2000	Manual	24	6 mo	Responders: 21.8% Partial: 26% None: 52%
Radmayr and colleagues	2001	Laser	20	6 mo	Responders: 65% Partial: 26% None: 5%
Serel and colleagues	2001	Manual	50	13 mo	Responders: 80% None: 6%
Honjo and colleagues	2002	Manual	15	2 mo	Responders: 47% None: 53%
Heller and colleagues	2004	Laser	24	3 mo	Responders: 25%

incontinence secondary to chronic spinal cord injury treated with acupuncture, reported a significant increase in the average maximum cystometric bladder capacity, achieving 38% cure rate and 38% symptom improvements [13].

The exact mechanism by which acupuncture exerts its therapeutic role on the bladder or nervous system is not clear. The noradrenergic neurons in the pontine locus coeruleus, an important supraspinal micturition center, control the sacral parasympathetic micturition center located in the intermediolateral nucleus in the sacral spinal cord by a descending noradrenergic pathway. Dopamine can act on the dopaminergic receptors in the pontine locus coeruleus, increasing synthesis of dopamine β-hydroxylase (responsible for noradrenalin synthesis), and on the cholinergic neurons in the sacral micturition center, increasing synthesis of choline acetyltransferase (responsible for acetylcholine synthesis). The end result is inducing bladder hyperactivity.

Wang and colleagues [14] showed that by injecting ι-dopa, a dopamine precursor, intraperitoneally to induce bladder hyperactivity in rats, the levels of dopamine β-hydroxylase (DBH) and choline acetyltransferase (ChAT) have increased significantly in the pontine locus coeruleus and the sacral intermediolateral nucleus, respectively, compared with control rats injected with saline. Furthermore, electroacupunture of point Zhonglushu (B29) has resulted in decreased micturition, basal bladder pressure, DBH levels, and ChAT levels, indicating that electroacupuncture inhibited ι-dopa–induced bladder hyperactivity by suppressing the excessively excited pontine and sacral micturition centers, thereby suppressing release of noradrenalin and acetylcholine from both centers, respectively. These investigators concluded that the effect of acupuncture depended mainly on supraspinal micturition centers.

In a group of children treated with electroacupuncture for primary nocturnal enuresis, 50% of parents noted that it was easier to waken their children in the morning [8]. Animal studies indicate that the pontine locus coeruleus has a key role in initiating cortical arousal to many stimuli, including bladder distension [15]. This may suggest that electroacupuncture, by influencing the noradrenergic projection from the locus coeruleus, which in turn increases the production of vasopressin, plays a role in the observation of decreased sleep arousal threshold and polyuria seen in this cohort of children. Investigators have used different adjunct techniques with the traditional manual acupuncture, including slow electric current and laser stimulation with various success rates. Although some authors suggested superior outcomes using electric stimulation, this was not apparently the case (see Table 1). It also has been suggested that acupuncture was more successful in preadolescent and adolescent children compared with younger children [10,11].

Acupuncture seemed to be well tolerated by most children, with no documented serious side effects. Few investigators, however, have reported on relapse rates after discontinuing acupuncture therapy sessions. Serel and colleagues [11] reported 80% success rate with a relapse rate of only 5% in a cohort of 50 children who had persistent primary nocturnal enuresis treated with traditional manual Chinese acupuncture and followed for 13 months.

In summary, acupuncture seems to be an attractive alternative therapeutic modality to conventional therapies in selected children with primary nocturnal enuresis.

Posterior tibial nerve stimulation

In 1983, McGuire and colleagues [16] were the first to report experience with posterior tibial nerve stimulation (PTNS) as an alternative therapeutic modality in treating patients who had urinary urgency secondary to detrusor instability with good results. Thereafter, several studies have evaluated PTNS efficacy as a neuromodulator in the treatment of a variety of lower urinary tract symptoms (LUTS) with various results.

The posterior tibial nerve is a mixed nerve that contains fibers originating from the same spinal segments as the parasympathetic innervation to the bladder, namely L5–S2 [17]. The procedure is performed by percutaneously inserting a 34-gauge stainless steel needle three fingerbreadths above the medial malleolus, between the posterior margin of the tibia and the soleus muscle. A stick-on electrode is placed on the same leg near the arch of the foot. The needle and electrode are connected to a low-voltage (9 V) stimulator with an adjustable pulse intensity of 0 to 10 mA. A fixed pulse width of 200 microseconds and a frequency of 20 Hz then are used [18]. Electrical stimulation of the posterior tibial nerve will result in a sensory response (tickling sensation in the sole of the foot) as well as a motor response, typically plantar flexion of the big toe or fanning of all toes. Treatment sessions usually are given weekly with each lasting approximately 30 minutes.

PTNS has proved effective and well tolerated among adults, but little has been published about the role of PTNS in the treatment of refractory LUTS among children. It is believed that the invasiveness of the procedure is responsible for its poor diffusion among pediatric urologists. Tanagho [19] reported the initial pediatric experience with PTNS in 1992; two recent reports have described PTNS' role in the pediatric population. De Gennaro [20] and colleagues reported their experience in the tolerability of PTNS among 23 children who had refractory nonneurogenic LUTS. Among children who had overactive bladder they observed 80% symptom improvement, with 44% of children achieving complete dryness and 62.5% achieving normalization of cystometric bladder capacity. Seventy-one percent of the group with nonneurogenic urinary retention had improvement. Nevertheless, none of the children who had neurogenic bladder had symptom improvement. They found the procedure to be safe and minimally painful.

Similarly, Hoebeke and colleagues [21], in a prospective cohort study of 32 children who had mixed LUTS resistant to conventional therapy, observed disappearance of urinary urgency in 7 of 28 children and improvement in 10. Four of the children who had daytime incontinence before treatment became completely dry and incontinence decreased in 12. Furthermore, these authors observed an overall statistically significant increase in mean bladder capacity among the group.

PTNS is a viable option in treating selected children with a variety of LUTS, but more studies are needed to better clarify its effectiveness and tolerability among pediatric population.

Transurethral electric bladder stimulation

Transurethral electric bladder stimulation (TEBS) is a technique based on biofeedback stimulation of insensate bladders. The goal of this neuromodulation modality is to allow children who have neurogenic bladder secondary to spinal cord injury or spinal dysraphism to recognize bladder filling and initiate volitional voiding, enabling children to become continent while storing urine in a low-pressure reservoir.

The technique involves filling the bladder partially with saline and then placing a special electrocatheter transurethrally. After a ground is placed in an arm or leg, the bladder is stimulated through the active electrode in the electrocatheter. One port is used to record intravesical pressure while patients simultaneously observe an attached water manometer to detect changes in bladder pressure. When the bladder begins to respond to stimulation, the patient senses a faint urge as tingling or burning in the bladder region, and a small bladder contraction of 3 to 5 cm H_2O is observed. With more sessions of TEBS, the amplitude of detrusor contractions increases, and the urge is stronger. Ultimately, incontinent patients who perceive the urge sensations will be able to stop bladder contraction by straining, and patients who have urinary retention begin to void with decreasing postvoid residuals [22].

Katana and Bereny [23] first introduced TEBS in Hungary in 1958. One hundred children who had meningomyelocele were treated between 1958 and 1975. Volitional day and night control were achieved in 71% of the children. Despite using the exact technique described by Katana and Bereny, no investigators in Europe or North America were able to duplicate their successes. Madersbacher and colleagues [24] reported on 30 patients with incomplete spinal cord injuries achieving urinary control in 56% of the patients. It is difficult to predict the nature of bladder recovery in patients who have partial spinal cord injury; therefore, lack of a comparable control group to determine if a statistical significant difference would be found in the untreated group is considered a drawback in their study.

Kaplan and Richards [25] deserve credit for introducing TEBS in North America in 1984. Their initial experience was published in 1986. All 24 recruited patients developed significant detrusor contractions, and in four, this was accompanied by urge to urinate. Their second reported series involved 62 patients; 21 completed three series of TEBS, and 38% of those voided with total control [26]. Furthermore, they observed that TEBS stimulated growth of bladder capacity to match that of normal children. This was reflected in a multi-institutional trial involving 11 different centers; the records of 335 children were available to study the role of TEBS in relation to bladder capacity and compliance before and after treatment. Fifty-three percent of patients had increased bladder capacity by 20% or greater after treatment. Furthermore, in 90% of patients, intravesical pressure was decreased or maintained within a safe range of less than 40 cm H_2O [27].

In another North American study, Decter and colleagues [28] observed an increase in age-adjusted bladder capacity in 33% and a decrease in end-filling pressures in 28% of 25 patients followed for 4 years. They stated, "the urodynamic improvements we achieved after stimulation did not alter the daily voiding routine (ie, clean intermittent catheterization) of these children."

Reviewing the available data, one can observe the conflicting results since TEBS was introduced by Katona. Most children studied have compromised innervated bladders, both with respect to peripheral afferent and efferent pathways and to micturition centers in the brain stem. A recent study from Sweden recruited 44 children, 24 who had idiopathic underactive bladder and 20 who had neurogenic underactive bladder, to receive TEBS as an alternative to clean intermittent catheterization (CIC). Thirty-nine children completed the study. After 2.5 years of follow-up, 83% and 40% of the children who had idiopathic and neurogenic underactive bladders achieved normalization of voiding, respectively. Of those on CIC, 73% succeeded in discontinuing catheterization [29]. The investigators concluded that TEBS is a promising method to treat the underactive detrusor in children. Their study avoided

biofeedback input during treatment sessions among children, a concept that was emphasized repeatedly by the originator of the technique to achieve successful outcomes. The investigators attributed failure of other earlier studies to demonstrate good outcomes to either not using higher current intensities or exclusively recruiting patients without control for preserved nerve functions, as is clear from their superior outcome in the group with idiopathic underactive bladders. In another recently conducted study, Han and colleagues [30] observed a concomitant improvement in fecal incontinence among children with spinal dyraphism undergoing TEBS to decrease uninhibited bladder contractions and increase bladder capacity or bladder sensation.

TEBS seems to be a promising alternative neuromodulator in selected patients. Given the limitations in conducting trials using TEBS (secondary to its time consumption for caregivers and parents and the need for highly skilled physicians, nurses, and therapists), it is hoped that trials recruiting larger numbers of patients from multiple centers with longer follow-ups will prepare the ground for TEBS in the future and highlight its value as an alternative to conventional therapeutic modalities in children who have voiding dysfunction.

Sacral nerve root stimulation

Sacral nerve root stimulation (SNS) was first approved in the United States for use in adults who have urge incontinence in September 1997. Since then, the indications have been broadened to include urgency-frequency syndrome and non-obstructive urinary retention. Additionally, this technology has been applied with various success to interstitial cystitis, pelvic pain syndromes, and fecal incontinence. The reversible implantable device, InterStim (Medtronic, Minneapolis, Minnesota), has been tested largely in adults with impressive functional results and symptomatic relief, depending on the series. There has been a lack of reported data addressing the efficiency of or complications associated with this device in the pediatric population, however.

DES represents a broad spectrum of functional disturbances involving the urinary and lower gastrointestinal (GI) systems in the absence of urologic anomalies or obvious neurologic disease [31]. The anatomic proximity, the common embryologic origin (endoderm), and the shared innervations (sacral pelvic plexus) of the urinary and

GI systems tend to link them. It is common for pediatric patients who have voiding dysfunctions (eg, incontinence, urgency, frequency, posturing) also to have associated defecation abnormalities (eg, encopresis, constipation, or fecal retention). Often the resolution of the voiding dysfunction depends on comanagement of the defecation abnormalities. Once a complete medical history, physical examination, and tests have ruled out other etiologies of elimination dysfunction, the child may be diagnosed with DES by exclusion.

Several authors reported on the use of transcutaneous electric nerve stimulation (TENS) of S3 as a noninvasive neuromodulation modality in children who have LUTS resistant to conventional therapy. The device for TENS consists of the pulse generator with amplifier and electrodes. Electrodes are placed bilaterally on the skin overlying the level of S3, which is at the level of the greater sciatic notch, one fingerbreadth lateral to the midline spinosus processus. Using this technique, Hoebeke and colleagues [32] observed 76% response rate with an increase in bladder capacity and a decrease in urgency and urge incontinence in 41 children who had detrusor hyperactivity treated with TENS. After 1 year of follow-up, relapse was noted in seven children, leaving 21 of 41 children (51.2%) definitively cured. Similarly, a 73.3% improved dryness with significant increase in mean voided volume also was reported by Bower and colleagues [33] in a cohort of 17 children treated for urinary urgency or urge incontinence.

To our knowledge, no data exist on the use of InterStim in the pediatric population. The perceived invasiveness of placing electrodes percutaneously into sacral foramina is probably the most important factor associated with its poor diffusion in the pediatric population.

The technique involves placing the patient in the prone position under general anesthesia. A spinal needle is inserted percutaneously into S3 foramina under fluoroscopic guidance. Once adequate positioning is confirmed with electrostimulation (visualization of the bellows motor response: a pulling down movement of the anal verge, flexion of ipsilateral first toe) the needle is removed, leaving the outer sheath in situ. A stimulating wire then can be passed down the sheath deep to the inner table of the bone, maintaining a coupling with the nerve. The outer sheath is removed, and a tunneled subcutaneous extender connecting the lead to an external pulse generator for programming is placed to begin the trial SNS period, which lasts 3 to 4 weeks. If successful, the patient will undergo a second procedure to implant the permanent InterStim neurostimulator device into the upper gluteal region [34].

Recently, the authors presented their experience with the InterStim device in the treatment of 23 children with various LUTS [35]. Between April 2001 and December 2003, 19 girls (mean age 11.1 years) and four boys (mean age 10.2 years) underwent SNS with the InterStim system.

All patients underwent a detailed medical history and physical examination. Additionally, each patient had a urine analysis and culture, plain abdominal radiograph, upper-tract ultrasonography, and uroflow with a residual urine check or complete urodynamic evaluation to rule out other potential etiologies of their DES. All families were required to maintain a urinary and defecation diary before and after therapeutic intervention. To qualify for InterStim therapy, families and patients were required to demonstrate a high level of motivation and were tried on at least 6 months of maximal medical therapy and behavioral modification before undergoing a trial of SNS therapy. A database was maintained to document symptoms (urinary leakage, nighttime leakage, urinary tract infections, urgency, frequency, posturing, constipation, discomfort with urination or defecation, urinary retention), family history, attempted therapy (behavior modification, dietary changes, biofeedback, intermittent catheterization, bowel program, medications), results during temporary neuromodulation, results after permanent neurostimulator placement, and overall patient and caregiver satisfaction with the therapy at their most recent clinic visit.

Of the 24 patients who underwent a trial period of SNS, 21 (88%) met the criteria for permanent InterStim device placement. Three patients were explanted: one was excluded secondary to cerebral palsy, one never turned the device on for fear of electrocution, and one failed to have at least a 50% improvement in symptoms. Eighty-three percent (19/23) of patients complained of urinary incontinence pretreatment, which completely resolved in 16% (3/19), improved in 63% (12/19), or was unchanged in 21% (4/19) of patients after InterStim placement. Nocturnal enuresis was an initial complaint in 74% (17/23) of the patients and improved in 65% (11/17) and was unchanged in 35% (6/17) of patients. One patient developed overflow incontinence and nocturnal enuresis after permanent device placement. Of the 15 patients who had preoperative urinary retention, 60% (9/15) were improved after surgery. Preoperatively six patients were on intermittent catheterization three to four times per day. Thirty-three percent (2/6) no longer require CIC, whereas 67% (4/6) remain on self-catheterization. Of these four patients, one was explanted for fear of electrocution, two decreased their frequency of catheterization to before bedtime and twice per day, and one had to catheterize more frequently than before. Seventy-eight percent (18/23) of patients had at least one urinary tract infection (UTI) before treatment; only six (33%) patients developed a UTI postoperatively within the first year of follow-up. Bladder pain, urinary urgency, frequency, and constipation improved in 67% (8/12), 75% (12/16), 85% (11/13), and 77% (13/17) of patients, respectively. The number of medications required per patient before the procedure was 4.5, which decreased by an average of 3.0 medications per patient to 1.5 after surgery.

The overall patient and caregiver satisfaction rates were assessed and recorded. An average satisfaction rate of 60% for patients and 65% for caregivers was demonstrated after InterStim placement. The most common feedback from families was that the patient's symptoms were more improved during the trial SNS period than after the permanent device placement.

The procedures were well tolerated. Two quadrapolar sacral leads were explanted from the 23 patients for a total implant rate of 91%. The only complications encountered were a seroma anterior to the neurostimulator device, a brief episode of skin sensitivity over the device site, two neurostimulator device failures, and one lead that required revision. The overall complication rate, excluding explantation, was 22% (5/23).

The authors believe that SNS in children is a viable option for carefully selected patients who have failed other forms of therapy. SNS effectively and safely improves multiple quality of life issues in most patients who have DES. These patients are drier, have fewer irritable voiding symptoms, and have improved constipation. In addition, many require significantly fewer medications for control of their symptoms. Longer follow-up and meticulous data collection is needed before widespread application of this technology is appropriate for children.

Summary

Several neuromodulatory options are available for selected children who have voiding dysfunction resistant to conventional therapy. Integral to all types of treatment is an educated team that reinforces progress rather than cure and encourages long-term behavioral changes.

References

[1] Baozhu S, Xiyou W. Short-term effect in 135 cases of enuresis treated by wrist ankle needling. J Trad Chin Med 1985;5:27–8.
[2] Chunpu Y. Acupuncture of Guanyuan (Ren 4) and Baihui (DU 20) in treatment of 500 cases of enuresis. J Trad Chin Med 1988;8:197.
[3] Baoqin X. 302 cases of enuresis treated with acupuncture. J Trad Chin Med 1991;11:121–2.
[4] deJonge DA. Epidemiology of enuresis: survey of the literature. In: Kolvin I, Mackeith RC, Meadow SR, editors. Bladder control and enuresis. London: Heine-mann; 1973. p. 39–46.
[5] Forsythe WI, Redmond A. Enuresis and spontaneous cure rate: study of 1129 enuretics. Arch Dis Child 1974;49:259–63.
[6] Rushton HG. Nocturnal enuresis: epidemiology, evaluations and currently available treatment options. J Pediatr 1989;114:691–6.
[7] Hellstrom A-L, Hanson E, Hansson S, et al. Micturition habits and incontinence in 7-year-old Swedish school entrants. Eur J Pediatr 1990;149:434–7.
[8] Bjorkstrom G, Hellstrom AL, Andersson S. Electro-acupuncture in the treatment of children with mono-symptomatic nocturnal enuresis. Scand J Urol Nephrol 2000;34(1):21–6.
[9] Radmayr C, Schlager A, Studen M, et al. Prospective randomized trial using laser acupuncture versus desmopressin in the treatment of nocturnal enuresis. Eur Urol 2001;40(2):201–5.
[10] Honjo H, Kawauchi A, Ukimura O, et al. Treatment of monosymptomatic nocturnal enuresis by acupuncture: a preliminary study. Int J Urol 2002; 9(12):672–6.
[11] Serel TA, Perk H, Koyuncuoglu HR, et al. Acupuncture therapy in the management of persistent primary nocturnal enuresis-preliminary results. Scand J Urol Nephrol 2001;35(1):40–3.
[12] Heller G, Langen PH, Steffens J. Laser acupuncture as third-line therapy for primary nocturnal enuresis: first results of a prospective study [in German]. Urologe A 2004;43(7):803–6
[13] Honjo H, Kitakoji H, Kawakita K, et al. Acupuncture for urinary incontinence in patients with chronic spinal cord injury. A preliminary report. Nippon Hinyokika Gakkai Zasshi 1998;89(7):665–9.
[14] Wang S, Wang X. The inhibitory effect of acupuncture on L-dopa-induced hyperactivity of rat's bladder. International Congress Series 2002;1238:171–7.
[15] Page ME, Akaoka H, Aston-Jones G, et al. Bladder distension activates noradrenergic locus coeruleus neurons by an excitatory amino acid mechanism. Neuroscience 1992;51:555–63.

[16] McGuire EJ, Shi-Chun Z, Horwinski ER, et al. Treatment of motor and sensory detrusor instability by electrical stimulation. J Urol 1983;129:78–9.

[17] Vandonick V, Van Balken MR, Finazzi Agro E, et al. Posterior tibial nerve stimulation in the treatment of voiding dysfunction: urodynamic data. Neurourol Urodyn 2004;23:246–51.

[18] Van Balken MR, Vandoninck V, Gisolf KW, et al. Posterior tibial nerve stimulation as neuromodulative treatment of lower urinary tract dysfunction. J Urol 2001;166:914–8.

[19] Tanagho EA. Neuromodulation in the management of voiding dysfunction in children. J Urol 1992;148: 655–7.

[20] De Gennaro M, Capitanucci ML, Silveri MM, et al. Percutaneous tibial nerve neuromodulation is well tolerated in children and effective for treating refractory vesical dysfunction. J Urol 2004;171:1911–3.

[21] Hoebeke P, Renson C, Petillon L, et al. Percutaneous electrical nerve stimulation in children with therapy resistant nonneuropathic bladder sphincter dysfunction: a pilot study. J Urol 2002;168:2605–8.

[22] Decter RM. Intravesical electrical stimulation of the bladder: con. Urology 2000;56:5–8.

[23] Katona F. Intravescalis elektromos ingerles a hugyholyagbenulasok diagnosticajaban es therapiajaban. Idegzyogy Szle 1959;11:165.

[24] Madersbacher H, Pauer W, Reiner E, et al. Rehabilitation of micturition in patients with incomplete spinal cord lesions by transurethral electrostimulation of the bladder. Eur Urol 1982;8:111–6.

[25] Kaplan WE, Richards I. Intravesical transurethral electrotherapy for the neurogenic bladder. J Urol 1986;136:243–6.

[26] Kaplan WE, Richards I. Intravesical bladder stimulation in myelodysplasia. J Urol 1988;140:1282–4.

[27] Cheng EY, Richards I, Balcon A, et al. Bladder stimulation therapy improves bladder compliance: results from a multi-institutional trial. J Urol 1996; 156:761–4.

[28] Decter RM, Snyder P, Laudermilch C. Transurethral electrical stimulation: a followup report. J Urol 1994;152:812–4.

[29] Gladh G, Mattsson S, Lindstrom S. Intravesical stimulation in the treatment of micturition dysfunction in children Neurourol Urodyn 2003;22:233–42.

[30] Han SW, Kim MJ, Kim JH, et al. Intravesical electrical stimulation improves neurogenic bowel dysfunction in children with spina bifida. J Urol 2004;171:2648–50.

[31] Feng WC, Churchill BM. Dysfunctional elimination syndrome in children without obvious spinal cord diseases. Pediatr Clin North Am 2001;48:1489–504.

[32] Hoebeke P, Van Laecke E, Everaert K, et al. Transcutaneous neuromodulation for the urge syndrome in children: a pilot study. J Urol 2001;166:2416–9.

[33] Bower WF, Moore KH, Adams RD. A pilot study of the home application of transcutaneous neuromodulation in children with urgency or urge incontinence. J Urol 2001;166:2420–2.

[34] Seigel SW. Management of voiding dysfunction with an implantable neuroprosthesis. Urol Clin North Am 1992;19:163–70.

[35] Humphreys MR, Hollatz P, Reinberg YE, et al. Sacral neuromodulation in children: preliminary results in 16 patients. Paper presented at: Annual Meeting of the American Urological Association; May 8–13, 2004; San Francisco, CA.

ELSEVIER
SAUNDERS

Urol Clin N Am 32 (2005) 109–112

**UROLOGIC
CLINICS
of North America**

The *Bion* Device: A Minimally Invasive Implantable Ministimulator for Pudendal Nerve Neuromodulation in Patients with Detrusor Overactivity Incontinence

J.L.H.R. Bosch, MD, PhD

Department of Urology, University Medical Center Utrecht, PO Box 85500, Utrecht 3508 GA, The Netherlands

Sacral nerve neuromodulation using the Interstim device (Medtronic, Minneapolis, Minnesota) is a valuable treatment option in patients who have refractory detrusor overactivity incontinence [1]. The author has reported success rates of 86% and 60% after 6 and 47 months, respectively, in a group of 45 patients who had refractory detrusor overactivity incontinence [2]. Similar long-term success rates have been reported by other groups [3–5]. In the referred studies, success was defined as an improvement of 50% or more in the number of incontinence episodes or the number of pads used per day. Patients qualified for permanent implantation of a sacral foramen electrode coupled to a pulse generator after a successful subchronic percutaneous nerve evaluation (PNE) of the S3 spinal nerve. The PNE success rate is approximately 54% to 68% [1]. Recent experience with the staged implant techniques using a tined lead has resulted in a higher implantation rate of up to 80% in 15 patients with various indications [6–7]. Nonetheless, many patients who have detrusor overactivity incontinence do not respond to sacral nerve neuromodulation.

Data generated during clinical neurophysiologic studies may provide an explanation for these observations. It is assumed that sacral nerve neuromodulation works by inhibition of the voiding reflex as a result of electrical stimulation of sensory afferent fibers. Many of the sensory afferent nerve fibers contained in the sacral spinal nerves originate in the pudendal nerve. Furthermore, electrical stimulation of the dorsal nerve of the penis, which is a purely sensory branch of the pudendal nerve, can inhibit the voiding reflex [8]. Thus pudendal nerve afferents are particularly important for the inhibitory effect on the voiding reflex.

Pudendal afferent activity mapping during neurosurgical procedures of the sacral nerve roots has shown that the S1, S2, and S3 roots contribute 4%, 60.5%, and 35.5%, respectively, of the overall pudendal afferent activity [9]. Although S2 carries more pudendal afferents, the S3 spinal nerve is used preferentially for neuromodulatory purposes. S3 stimulation causes less unavoidable and undesired excitation of efferent fibers that innervate leg muscles compared with S2 stimulation. Pudendal afferent distribution, however, also is confined to a single level (ie, S2) in 18% or to a single root in 7.6% of cases [9]. A lack of effect of S3 stimulation therefore can be expected in at least 18% of cases.

Chronic pudendal nerve stimulation may be an alternative option in these patients. Direct pudendal nerve neuromodulation stimulates more afferents than S3 stimulation and therefore also may be more effective in those who have a significant contribution of pudendal afferents to S3. *Bion*-r therapy (Advanced Bionics Corp., Valencia, California) for pudendal nerve stimulation is a new minimally invasive option for effective neuromodulation.

The *bion*-r device

The *bion*-r (rechargeable bion) device is a self-contained, battery-powered, telemetrically

---

The author has been principal investigator of the *bion*-r pilot study that was sponsored by Advanced Bionics Corp., Valencia, California.

E-mail address: ruudbosc@euronet.nl

programmable, current-controlled minineurosti-mulator with an integrated electrode. It is 27 mm × 3.3 mm in size and weighs 0.7 g. It can be implanted adjacent to the pudendal nerve at Alcock's canal. A previous prototype, the radio-frequency-activated bion (RF-bion) did not have an integrated battery and used an external radio-frequency-transmitting coil that provided power and commanded the implanted RF-bion [10]. The external components of that neural prosthesis had to be worn in a belt around the subject's waist.

Percutaneous screening test

Subjects qualify for implantation after a positive percutaneous screening test (PST), which includes the performance of a cystometrogram without and with percutaneous pudendal nerve stimulation. The ischial spine is a good landmark of the site where the pudendal nerve reenters the pelvis and Alcock's canal. After local anesthesia of the skin, the stimulating needle is advanced through the ischial rectal fossa. The correct site for stimulation is located using vaginal palpation of the ischial spine and electrodiagnosis. X-ray screening also may be helpful if available. The pudendal nerve is stimulated through the stimulating needle (12.5 cm, 20 gauge) and an external pulse generator with the following parameter settings: frequency 20 Hz, pulse width 200 microseconds, duty cycle 50% (4.92 seconds on/4.92 seconds off). The amplitude, maximally 10 mA, is adjusted to the patient's sensations. A second cystometrogram is performed after 10 minutes of stimulation. A PST is consid-ered positive if stimulation results in a more than 50% increase in the bladder volume at the first involuntary detrusor contraction or the maximum cystometric capacity. The test is repeated at the contralateral side in case of a negative result.

Implantation procedure

After a successful PST the *bion*-r can be implanted at its target location, adjacent to the pudendal nerve at Alcock's canal. Implantation is performed with a specially developed toolkit after making a 2- to 3-mm skin incision 1.5 cm medial to the ischial tuberosity. One of the parts of the tool is a cylindrically shaped sheath, the so-called "introducer." In this sheath, a blunt-tipped dis-sector/stimulator is placed. This device is ad-vanced through the ischial rectal fossa while vaginally palpating the ischial spine. Palpation of the ischial spine, x-ray screening, and electro-diagnosis again are used for guidance of the

implant tool. The blunt dissector stimulator is connected to an external pulse generator to identify the optimal position where the stimulat-ing current produces a visual contraction of the paravaginal muscles or the anal sphincter and sometimes of the levator ani. The patient may report a sensory response in the vaginal, vulvar, clitoridal, and perianal area. Compound muscle action potentials also may be recorded from the anal sphincter. The blunt dissector/stimulator then is removed, keeping the introducer sheath in exactly the same place. The bion, held in the tip of the bion holder, is advanced through the introducer. In this way the bion is placed in the exact spot where a typical pudendal response was achieved during stimulation. The bion now is positioned using the placement device that with-draws the plastic sheath that surrounds the bion. The tool, consisting of introducer, bion holder, and placement device, is removed, leaving the bion in the desired position (Fig. 1).

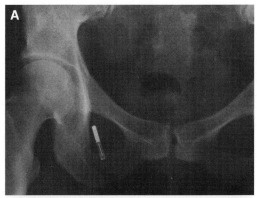

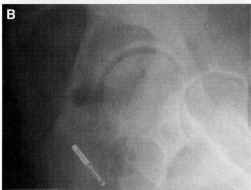

Fig. 1. (*A*) Antero-posterior radiograph of the pelvis with the bion in position close to Alcock's canal. (*B*) Lateral radiograph of the pelvis with bion device parallel to the pudendal nerve in Alcock's canal.

The implantations take place in an operating room with the patient sedated but able to communicate with the surgeon and the skin locally anaesthetized.

Postimplantation management

The device is activated 8 to 14 days after implantation. The physician programs the bion through radiofrequency telemetry signals. Specially developed software and a system of communication comprised of the recharging system, base station, and chair pad are used to program the appropriate stimulation parameters. The default stimulation parameters are as described previously. Unlike the discontinued RF-bion, the *bion*-r is a self-contained stimulator with an integrated battery. The lithium-ion battery needs to be recharged regularly, preferentially daily. To this end, the patient sits on a specially developed chair pad powered by a wall outlet. A remote control can be used to change the stimulation amplitude within a preset range and to turn the bion on or off. The physician can change the stimulation parameters and the allowed range of amplitudes using a programming system (base station). Voiding-incontinence diaries are used for the evaluation of therapy. The volume of urine voided per micturition, the number of incontinence episodes, and the number of pads used were recorded.

Pilot studies

RF-bion

The first RF-bion implantation was performed in August 2000 [10]. Of an unknown number of patients undergoing a PST, five female patients with overactive bladder symptoms responded with a 50% or more increase in maximum cystometric capacity. These women received an RF-bion implant. In PST-responders, the maximum cystometric capacity increased from 325 mL to 610 mL on average during the acute test. After a follow-up of 45 days, the number of incontinence episodes had decreased from an average of 3.5 to 1.5 per day and the number of incontinence pads decreased from an average of 4.3 to 1.4 per day [10].

Bion-*r*

The first *bion*-r implantation was performed in December 2002 [11]. The results from this pilot study of female patients who had refractory detrusor overactivity incontinence using the *bion*-r have been reported [11,12].

A PST was planned in 15 women who had idiopathic urodynamically demonstrated detrusor overactivity incontinence and who had failed drug treatment, pelvic floor physiotherapy, and various forms of neuromodulation, including vaginal plug stimulation, posterior tibial nerve stimulation, and sacral nerve stimulation. In one patient, detrusor overactivity could not be confirmed during the baseline cystometrogram. Of the 14 remaining patients, five responded to the PST and received a *bion*-r implant.

Voiding diary parameters showed that the average volume voided per micturition increased moderately, but the voiding frequency decreased. This indicates that treatment effects were not caused by a change in drinking behavior.

After 6 months of follow-up the average number of incontinence episodes had decreased from 6.9 to 2.9 per day and the average volume voided per micturition had increased moderately from 139 to 154 mL [12]. Urodynamic studies after 6 months compared with baseline revealed an average increase of maximum cystometric capacity from 272 to 419 mL [11].

Given that four of five patients previously had failed sacral nerve neuromodulation, a 57% decrease in the number of incontinence episodes compares favorably to the 6-months results obtained in a group of 36 refractory urge incontinence patients treated with S3 sacral nerve neuromodulation in the author's institution [13]. The latter patients on average had a 72% decrease in the number of incontinence episodes.

Summary

The results of the bion pilot studies indicate that a considerable reduction in the degree of detrusor overactivity incontinence can be obtained in severely refractory cases, including women who had failed sacral nerve neuromodulation. The described technique is well tolerated by the patients. It is minimally invasive and relatively simple. Clinical trials of the *bion*-r device involving larger numbers of patients are underway in the United States and Europe. A subchronic instead of the currently used acute screening test might increase the percentage of patients assessed as suitable candidates for implantation. Therefore, methods of performing a subchronic test of the pudendal nerve also are being investigated.

References

[1] Bosch JLHR, Groen J. Sacral nerve neuromodulation in the treatment of refractory motor urge incontinence. Curr Opin Urol 2001;11: 399–403.

[2] Bosch JLHR, Groen J. Sacral nerve neuromodulation in the treatment of patients with refractory motor urge incontinence: long-term results of a prospective longitudinal study. J Urol 2000;163: 1219–22.

[3] Siegel SW, Catanzaro F, Dijkema HE, et al. Long-term results of a multicenter study on sacral nerve stimulation for treatment of urinary urge incontinence, urgency-frequency, and retention. Urology 2000;56(Suppl 6A):87–91.

[4] Janknegt RA, Hassouna MM, Siegel SW, et al. Long-term effectiveness of sacral nerve stimulation for refractory urge incontinence. Eur Urol 2001;39: 101–6.

[5] Spinelli M, Bertapelle P, Cappellano F, et al. De Seta F on behalf of the GINS group: chronic sacral neuromodulation in patients with lower urinary tract symptoms: results from a national register. J Urol 2001;166:541–5.

[6] Spinelli M, Giardello G, Gerber M, et al. New sacral neuromodulation lead for percutaneous implantation using local anesthesia: description and first experience. J Urol 2003;170:1905–7.

[7] Spinelli M, Giardello G, Arduini A, et al. New percutaneous technique of sacral nerve stimulation has high initial success rate: preliminary results. Eur Urol 2003;43:70–4.

[8] Craggs M, Edhem I, Knight S, et al. Suppression of normal human voiding reflexes by electrical stimulation of the dorsal penile nerve. Eur Urol 1998; 33(Suppl):60. Abstract 239.

[9] Huang JC, Deletis V, Vodusek DB, et al. Preservation of pudendal afferents in sacral rhizotomies. Neurosurgery 1997;41:411–5.

[10] Grill WM, Craggs MD, Foreman RD, et al. Emerging clinical applications of electrical stimulation: opportunities for restoration of function. J Rehabil Res Dev 2001;38:641–53.

[11] Bosch R. Treatment of refractory urge urinary incontinence by a novel minimally invasive implantable pudendal nerve mini-stimulator. J Pelvic Med Surg 2003;9:310. Abstract 11.

[12] Bosch R, Groen J. Treatment of refractory urge urinary incontinence by a novel minimally invasive implantable pudendal nerve mini-stimulator. J Urol 2004;171(suppl 4):130. Abstract 488.

[13] Bosch R, Groen J. Complete 5-year follow-up of sacral (S3) segmental nerve stimulation with an implantable electrode and pulse generator in 36 consecutive patients with refractory detrusor overactivity incontinence. Neurourol Urodyn 2002;21: 390–1.

UROLOGIC
CLINICS
of North America

Urol Clin N Am 32 (2005) 113–115

Future Directions in Pelvic Neuromodulation

Firouz Daneshgari, MD[a],*, Paul Abrams, MD[b]

[a]Center for Female Pelvic Medicine and Reconstructive Surgery, Glickman Urological Institute,
Cleveland Clinic Foundation, 9500 Euclid Avenue, A100, Cleveland, OH 44195, USA
[b]Bristol Urological Institute, Southmead Hospital, Bristol BS10 5NB, United Kingdom

Peripheral neurologic control of the bladder via autonomic and somatic innervations to correct problematic bladder dysfunction has come a long way from its introduction in 1863, when Giannuzzi stimulated the spinal cord in dogs and concluded that the hypogastric and pelvic nerves are involved in regulation of the bladder (see the article by Fandel and Tanagho elsewhere in this issue). The first attempt at bladder stimulation occurred in 1878, when Saxtorph treated patients with urinary retention by way of intravesicle electrical stimulation [1]. After experimentations with various methods of stimulating the bladder— such as the transurethral approach, direct detrusor stimulation [2], pelvic nerve stimulation [3], pelvic floor stimulation [4], and spinal cord stimulation [5] built on the pioneering work of Tanagho and later Schmidt [6–9]—it was demonstrated that stimulation of sacral root S3 generally induces detrusor and sphincter action [9].

Finally, in October 1997, after two decades of experimentation with various approaches to sacral root stimulation, sacral neurostimulation (SNS) for treatment of refractory urge incontinence was approved by the US Food and Drug Administration in the United States. At the time of this writing, approximately 20,000 SNSs (Interstim. Metronic Inc., Minneapolis, MN) have been implanted worldwide. Since the approval of SNS in 1997, a number of technical advances have been made to reduce previous difficulties with the placement of a test lead or a permanent generator. However, trial and error continues to be the main approach for the selection of patients eligible for

SNS implantation. Little progress has been made to advance our understanding of the mechanism of action, and, more importantly, the predictors of outcome for patients who are eligible for SNS placement. Short of trying the procedure, we still do not have clinical criteria that will allow us to tell our patients whether they will be responsive to SNS stimulation.

In view of the success of SNS, new lines of research are enabling us to do more selective stimulation of the innervation of the bladder at more peripheral sites, such as pudendal nerve stimulation, and with the use of less invasive devices, such as Bion and other in situ implantable devices. The aim of this research is to determine if a less invasive, more selective stimulation or an event-driven (detrusor overactivity or a desire for micturition) [10] stimulus would allow for a more improved and durable response.

Looking forward to the future development of this field, we asked the contributing authors of this issue of the *Urologic Clinics of North America* to pose important research questions worth pursuing in the next few years. Below is a list of the selected topics, followed by the name of the contributing authors who suggested them:

1. Determining clinical predictors of responders versus nonresponders. It is highly desirable to predict—with a reasonable level of accuracy—the potential response of patients to SNS, thus avoiding the need for a test trial (Daneshgari).

   The above information may result from any of the following studies:

   a. A longitudinal prospective study of cohort patients with approved indications for SNS in whom the parameters of clinical,

* Corresponding author.
  E-mail address: daneshf@ccf.org (F. Daneshgari).

urodynamic, imaging (positron emission tomography or functional MRI), stimulation parameters, and other potential biomarkers (urine proteins, growth factors) are vigorously documented through stages of SNS and during a 2-year follow-up.

b. A case–control study of the previous recipients of SNS-staged implants, in which the predictive factors of positive responders (cases), and nonresponders (controls) could be studied.

2. Comparing the effects of continuous versus intermittent stimulation to test the acute vs. chronic (neural plasticity–mediated) mechanism of action for SNS (Daneshgari).

The above information will likely result from a prospective randomized clinical trial (RCT) of intermittent or continuous SNS in any of the approved indications.

3. Comparing the efficacy of peripheral nerve stimulation (PIN) with SNS in the treatment of refractory overactive bladders or frequency/urgency symptoms (Daneshgari).

4. Comparing the efficacy of SNS with pharmacologic therapy including anticholinergic/muscarinic receptor inhibitors (MRAs) in the treatment of refractory overactive bladders or frequency/urgency symptoms (Daneshgari).

The above information will likely result from a prospective RCT of SNS versus PIN versus MRAs for treatment of refractory overactive bladders or frequency/urgency.

5. Determining whether a unilateral versus bilateral stimulation in either category of the current indications would lead to an improved and more durable response (Daneshgari and Hassouna).

The above information will likely result from a prospective RCT of unilateral or bilateral SNS for any of the approved indications.

6. Determining the efficacy and durability of botulinum toxin A (Botox) for treatment of refractory overactive bladders (Daneshgari).

The above information will likely result from a prospective RCT comparing the effects of botulinum toxin versus placebo.

7. Determining the efficacy and durability of the use of SNS in patients with idiopathic constipation (Jarrett).

Given the ethical limitations for a nontreatment group, the above information will likely result from:

a. a prospective RCT between SNS and an existing standard of care for idiopathic constipation, or

b. a prospective cohort observational study of the use of SNS in patients with idiopathic constipation.

8. Determining the efficacy and durability of the use of SNS in patients with fecal incontinence secondary to obstetric damage (Jarrett).

The above information will likely result from a prospective observational study or an RCT to assess the effects of SNS against the currently available treatment.

9. Conducting a comparative trial of the effects of direct pudendal nerve stimulation versus SNS in patients with refractory overactive bladder (OAB) (Bosch).

The above information will result from a prospective RCT comparing the effects of pudendal nerve stimulation versus SNS in patients with refractory OAB.

10. Conducting functional brain imaging of SNS responders and nonresponders to study the CNS effects of SNS in these two groups (Bosch).

The above information will likely result from a prospective observational study of the recipients of stages of SNS (similar to question 2 above).

11. Conducting a prospective study to evaluate the timing of PIN for optimal long-term results (Stroller).

The above information will result from a prospective RCT comparing the effectiveness of the different lengths of PIN with a long-term follow-up.

12. Developing animal models to better delineate mechanisms of action for neuromodulation (ie, neurotransmitters) (Daneshgari and Stroller).

Use of animal models in the laboratory will allow us to investigate the effects of electrical stimulation on:

a. Cells, tissues, and organs such as nerves, pelvic floor musculature, bladder, vagina, and bowels.

b. The central nervous compartments involved in pelvic floor function.

13. Conducting a prospective observational study to investigate cross-organ effects of neuromodulation (SNS or peripheral stimulation) in patients with genitourinary, gastrointestinal, and gynecologic complaints (Stroller).

The above information will likely result from a prospective observational study of recipients of stages of SNS (similar to questions 2 and 8 above).

14. Determining the validity, accuracy, and reproducibility of electrophysiologic measurements for placement of SNS, to be followed by investigation of the association between the results of electrophysiologic measures and the length of positive response to SNS (Chai). The above information will likely result from a prospective observational study of recipients of stages of SNS (similar to questions 2, 8, and 11 above).

15. Devising studies to elucidate the precise pathophysiologic mechanisms for urge incontinence, and thereby the mechanism of action of SNS (Chai).

16. Using injectable agents such as botulinum toxin A in conjunction with SNS (as adjuvant or neoadjuvant therapy) to enhance the proportion of patients responsive to neuromodulatory treatment for their refractory overactive bladders (Hassouna).

   The above information will result from a prospective RCT comparing the effectiveness of mono-therapy (SNS) with that of SNS + botulinum toxin A injections.

17. Conducting studies to discover potential urinary biomarkers (such as a nerve growth factor) as a diagnostic tool to distinguish between potential responders and nonresponders (Hassouna).

   The above information may result from a longitudinal perspective study of cohort patients with approved indications for SNS in whom the parameters of clinical, urodynamic, imaging (pet scanning or functional MRI), stimulation parameters, and other potential biomarkers (urine proteins, growth factors)

are vigorously documented through stages of SNS and during a 2-year follow-up.

We hope that addressing some of the above questions in the coming years will allow us to enhance our understanding of the role of neuromodulation in treating the challenging clinical conditions facing us.

References

[1] Madersbacher H. Konservative Therapie der neurogenen Blasendysfunktion. Urologe A 1999;38:24–9.

[2] Boyce WH, Lathem JE, Hunt LD. Research related to the development of an artificial electrical stimulator for the paralyzed human bladder: a review. J Urol 1964;91:41–51.

[3] Dees JE. Contraction of the urinary bladder produced by electric stimulation. Preliminary report. Invest Urol 1965;2:539–47.

[4] Caldwell KP. The electrical control of sphincter incompetence. Lancet 1963;2:174–5.

[5] Nashold BS Jr, Friedman H, Boyarsky S. Electrical activation of micturition by spinal cord stimulation. J Surg Res 1971;11:144–7.

[6] Heine JP, Schmidt RA, Tanagho EA. Intraspinal sacral root stimulation for controlled micturition. Invest Urol 1977;15:78–82.

[7] Schmidt RA, Bruschini H, Tanagho EA. Urinary bladder and sphincter responses to stimulation of dorsal and ventral sacral roots. Invest Urol 1979; 16:300–4.

[8] Tanagho EA, Schmidt RA. Bladder pacemaker: scientific basis and clinical future. Urology 1982;20: 614–9.

[9] Tanagho EA. Neural stimulation for bladder control. Semin Neurol 1988;8:170–3.

[10] Hansen J, Fjorback MV, Media S, et al. Automatic event driven electrical stimulation for treatment of neurogenic detrusor overactivity in spinal cord injured patients. Neurourol Urodyn 2004;23:475–6.

ELSEVIER
SAUNDERS

Urol Clin N Am 32 (2005) 117–120

UROLOGIC
CLINICS
of North America

Index

Note: Page numbers of article titles are in **boldface** type.

doi:10.1016/S0094-0143(05)00010-8

Changing Your Address?

Make sure your subscription changes too! When you notify us of your new address, you can help make our job easier by including an exact copy of your Clinics label number with your old address (see illustration below.) This number identifies you to our computer system and will speed the processing of your address change. Please be sure this label number accompanies your old address and your corrected address—you can send an old Clinics label with your number on it or just copy it exactly and send it to the address listed below.

We appreciate your help in our attempt to give you continuous coverage. Thank you.

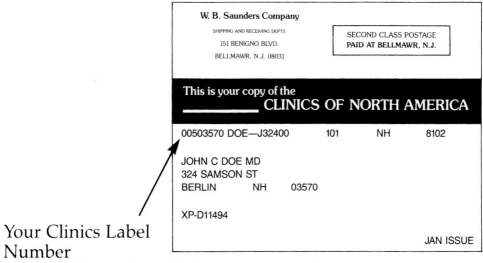

Your Clinics Label Number

Copy it exactly or send your label
along with your address to:
W.B. Saunders Company, Customer Service
Orlando, FL 32887-4800
Call Toll Free 1-800-654-2452

Please allow four to six weeks for delivery of new subscriptions and for processing address changes.